Stop
Inflammation
Now!

Stop
Inflam

A Step-by-Step

Plan to Prevent,

Treat, and Reverse

Inflammation—

the Leading Cause

of Heart Disease

and Related Conditions

mation
Now!

RICHARD M. FLEMING, M.D.

with TOM MONTE

AVERY

A MEMBER OF PENGUIN GROUP (USA) INC.

NEW YORK

Published by the Penguin Group
Penguin Group (USA) Inc., 375 Hudson Street, New York,
New York 10014, U.S.A. • Penguin Group (Canada), 10 Alcorn Avenue, Toronto,
Ontario M4V 3B2 Canada, (a division of Pearson Penguin Canada Inc.) • Penguin Books Ltd,
80 Strand, London WC2R 0RL, England • Penguin Ireland, 25 St. Stephen's Green, Dublin 2,
Ireland (a division of Penguin Books Ltd) • Penguin Books Australia Ltd, 250 Camberwell Road,
Camberwell, Victoria 3124, Australia (a division of Pearson Australia Group Pty Ltd) • Penguin
Books India Pvt Ltd, 11 Community Centre, Panchsheel Park, New Delhi–110 017, India •
Penguin Group (NZ), Cnr Airborne and Rosedale Roads, Albany, Auckland 1310, New Zealand
(a division of Pearson New Zealand Ltd) • Penguin Books (South Africa) (Pty) Ltd,
24 Sturdee Avenue, Rosebank, Johannesburg 2196, South Africa

Penguin Books Ltd, Registered Offices:
80 Strand, London WC2R 0RL, England
First Avery edition 2005
Copyright © 2004 by Richard M. Fleming, M.D., and Tom Monte

The Library of Congress cataloged the hardcover edition as follows:
Fleming, Richard M.
Stop inflammation now! : a step-by-step plan to prevent, treat, and reverse
inflammation—the leading cause of heart disease and related conditions /
Richard Fleming with Tom Monte.
p. cm.
Includes bibliographical references and index.
ISBN 0-399-15111-7
1. Inflammation—Popular works. 2. Coronary heart disease—Prevention—Popular
works. 3. Arteritis—Prevention—Popular works. I. Monte, Tom. II. Title.
RB131.F546 2004 2003046910
616'.0473—dc21

ISBN 1-58333-200-6 (paperback edition)

Printed in the United States of America
10 9 8 7 6 5 4 3 2 1

Book design by Tanya Maiboroda

Most Avery books are available at special quantity discounts for bulk purchase for sales promotions, premiums,
fund-raising, and educational needs. Special books or book excerpts also can be created to fit specific needs.
For details, write Penguin Group (USA) Inc. Special Markets, 375 Hudson Street, New York, NY 10014.

Contents

Acknowledgments

ALL AUTHORS recognize at some point the influence of people around them, people who are responsible in one way or another for their reaching the point where they have something of significance to write about. In my case, there are many people to thank. First, I would like to thank my parents, without whom I would not be here. Like many parents, they wanted the best for their children and hoped their children would indeed accomplish something. Next, I would like to thank my educators from elementary school and beyond, with a special nod to those from the seventh grade when I was placed in advanced science courses, as this gave me the opportunity to develop into a scientist. Third, I would like to thank my mentor and friend, Dr. Gordon Harrington, who encouraged me to pursue scientific truth and who helped hone my scientific and analytic abilities. I would like to thank both Stedman Mays and Mary Tahan (of the Clausen, Mays and Tahan Literary Agency), who believed in and worked to improve this book from its inception. Next, I would like to thank Tom Monte for his help in writing this book. I was tired of trying to understand why the practice of medicine lagged so far behind the science of medicine, tired of trying to publish many of these ideas in the medical literature, and there were many days when writing this book was the last thing I wanted to do. Through Tom's pen I was able to enjoy reading my own discoveries again, allowing me the opportunity to see my discoveries and theories in a fresh new light.

Of special interest to my family, our original meeting to discuss this book with agents and publishers was scheduled to take place in New York City on September 11, 2001. That meeting was canceled the Friday before because of an injury to someone we knew, who required hospitalization; all that could have happened to us as a result never occurred. Most important, I would like to thank my family: my children, who bring me joy and are quick to point out the flaws of many other diets, not to mention my own flaws, and finally, my wife, Diane.

Diane has stood beside me during periods of criticism and paid me the ultimate compliment when she said, "You know, you've been right for seventeen years." Lest the reader become confused, she meant "right" about the findings of my research during the last seventeen years and not about everything else. I dedicate this book to Diane, for she has put in the same seventeen years' worth of work. A long overdue thanks for her work, her sweat, her tears, and her *love.*

Foreword
Stop Inflammation Now!

YEARS AGO, former surgeon general C. Everett Koop said that eight out of ten leading causes of death in the United States were influenced by diet and lifestyle. Heart disease and coronary artery disease are without question the biggest killers of adults in this country. Even when heart disease doesn't kill, as a chronic disease with all its accompanying complications, physical limitations, and psychological effects, it certainly dampens one's lifestyle—that is, if it has been diagnosed. In addition, heart disease is an economic nightmare. It's a burden on the health-care system and on our own pocketbooks. Face it, heart disease costs us a lot and does so in a lot of ways.

A particular concern I have is that risk factors for heart disease are showing up in younger and younger people. Obesity is chief among these risk factors, and the prevalence of obesity among both adults and children has skyrocketed over the past 20 years. Indeed, according to Jeff Copeland, former head of the Centers for Disease Control and Prevention, "Obesity is as dramatic as anything I've seen in public health. . . . Obesity is the health problem of the century."

Obesity and heart disease risk, however, are strongly influenced by our diets and lifestyles, and that's a plus because it allows us some control over our health. Indeed, we really can do something about our weight and our health to minimize our risk of heart disease. To a certain extent, obesity and heart disease have some commonalities. They both take time to acquire (unless you were born with a congenital condition) and they are often influenced by lifestyle. Think about it: Gaining two pounds is not significant, but gaining two pounds every year for 20 years is very significant. Ditto with heart disease. A meal that is unfriendly to your heart is not a big deal. Combine 20 years of such meals with a sedentary life, however, and you're asking for trouble. In this way, obesity and heart disease are what I call "scorecard diseases." They reflect what's been happening for a long time. As such, they need a long-term solution, because a diet that lasts a week or two just isn't going to cut it.

Enter Dr. Richard Fleming. It's refreshing to see a book about reducing heart disease (perhaps even reversing many symptoms) written by a board-certified nuclear cardiologist. He points out how an important biomarker of heart disease—arterial inflammation—can be strongly influenced by diet and physical activity. He also defines this type of inflammation and how it impacts heart disease, and he does so in a clear, no-nonsense, and science-based way that consumers can understand. He's right—while inflammation has been a known risk factor for heart disease for some time, it has received too little credit for being the major player that it is.

Addressing serious chronic health problems requires a serious solution, and chronic arterial inflammation is no different. People with this type of inflammation and the cardiac profile that it brings with it need serious intervention—they need medical-nutrition therapy, a way of successfully managing nutrition-related health problems with nutritional intervention. Dr. Fleming's diet is just that—medical-nutrition therapy for people with heart disease. A casual experience it is not. Indeed, Dr. Fleming's diet and lifestyle plan may seem drastic at first, but so are the consequences of leaving heart disease untreated. Of course, he also points out that it can be extremely effective at reducing arterial inflammation.

The Fleming diet is primarily plant-based, but it does include very low-fat animal foods. It is high in fiber, and has plenty of fruits and vegetables, legumes, and whole-grain foods. In short, it has more of what most people's diets are missing. And it has many components that can reduce the risk for cancer. The creators of the National Cancer Institute's "Five-a-Day" program to promote more fruits and vegetables in the average American diet would love it if people ate as much produce as Dr. Fleming recommends. Indeed, five servings a day is very modest, and that number was never considered an ultimate goal for most adults. The emphasis is now on nine servings daily. If we had given these foods more attention throughout our earlier lives, and ate less of "the other stuff," then perhaps we wouldn't have nearly two out of three adults who are overweight and at a higher risk for heart disease, cancer, and other life-impeding conditions.

Dr. Fleming's plan, in its strictest form, is intended for those with serious heart disease who require serious medical-nutrition therapy, and it may not be everyone's cup of decaffeinated java, to be sure. As a dietetics professional who spends a lot of time counseling families about diet and lifestyle, I understand the importance of respecting people's decisions about these issues. Sorry, Richard, I'm the first one to declare that I'm not giving up my daily skim milk, eggs sometimes (their antioxidants taste too good), and the occasional piece of dark chocolate. And if I completely gave up olive oil, my family would feel betrayed, and their revenge would kill me faster than heart disease. These foods have served me well and I continue to enjoy good heart health. At the same time, I'm not giving up my mountain of fruits and vegetables, daily physical activity, meditation, and other lifestyle habits that complement my diet and support my health. For someone with acute heart disease who may be staring at a bypass, more drastic measures may be necessary than what is needed to maintain general prudent health.

No matter what positive changes in your diet and lifestyle you decide to make, be sure not to pass judgment until you give yourself a good four to six weeks to truly adapt to and assimilate the changes. You are acquiring new foods, tastes, and ways of living, and undoing years and layers of eating habits and lifestyles that may not have been friendly to your health. Even if you do not embrace Dr. Fleming's philosophy completely and follow it vigilantly, adopting even a milder version along with a more physically active lifestyle and some attention to stress-busting may improve your overall heart health. I often wonder how much better off Americans would be if, for instance, everyone ate just a few more fruits and vegetables and replaced a few refined grains with whole ones, threw in some legumes, and, of course, included some daily exercise. People would still eat "the other stuff" but less of it because there'd be less room for it. Imagine what 20 years of that kind of eating and living might do for us. It's still, ultimately, an individual decision, but in all my years of working with families, helping them to implement positive health and lifestyle changes, I never met anyone who regretted trying.

KEITH-THOMAS AYOOB, ED.D., R.D., FADA
Associate Professor
Albert Einstein College of Medicine

Introduction

GALILEO GALILEI SAID, "All truths are easy to understand once they are discovered. The point is to discover them." So it is with everything, including human health. When I first began my experience with the American Heart Association in 1976, it was believed that heart disease was the direct result of cholesterol, smoking, high blood pressure, obesity, lack of activity, being male, family history, and diabetes. Unfortunately, take medications, lose weight, stop smoking, or get other parents was where the advice tended to end. I was asked to become part of the physician cholesterol education faculty of the AHA, and we started working on cholesterol problems. We discovered that some people's cholesterol levels actually increased after they were placed on medication. Little attention was paid to the work by Ancel Keys and Nathan Pritikin, who both showed that diet was important in treating heart disease. These individuals were essentially ignored because they were not physicians, so what could they know! The truth is they knew a lot, because research done correctly is a better teacher than medicine or any school. During my training years I had the opportunity to be involved in research trying to reduce heart disease through dietary and lifestyle changes. Initially the numbers looked good, and the major criticism was how "difficult" it was for people to follow the recommended changes. Several years later I looked at most of the available information and discovered that lowering cholesterol alone resulted in only one third of the people getting better. Another one third got worse, and the remaining one third stayed the same. In other words, the results were *chance* and not anything we were doing! By 1994 I was disenchanted by our lack of progress. Our focus, it seemed, was more on adding medications and performing surgeries than on treating the underlying problem; we were treating the symptoms and not the cause.

Frustrated by the lack of better results, I took off my medical hat and returned to my scientific roots. I began asking the obvious questions: What are we missing, and why? By early 1995 I was looking at my data, as well as most of the information I could find about other researchers' work on heart disease. Every study was having some success, but no one was showing the results we were looking for. The answer behind why we weren't more successful was clear. We weren't working together, and no one wanted to credit their colleagues with anything. So researchers working on cholesterol ignored the work on homocysteine, and the homocysteine people ignored the work on fibrinogen, et cetera. The fight to determine who was right took precedence over finding the truth. Meanwhile, the emphasis on reducing fat in the diet resulted in everything becoming reduced-fat, which, in turn, lead to people eating more low-fat foods while at the same time eating more calories, forgetting that eating more calories can make people fat. America and the rest of the world suffered from more and more heart disease, diabetes, and obesity as a result. By 1995 I was incorporating all of these ideas into what would later become my unified theory of vascular disease. This would be ignored for the same reasons no one was working together to begin with: No one wanted to share credit for an idea, and everyone wanted complete credit for themselves. But the unified theory wasn't complete until June 1997. Several months earlier, I had listened to drug salesmen talk about a new drug for treating asthma. The medication was an interleukin inhibitor, and it worked by relaxing the smooth muscles in the airways of the lungs. And then it dawned on me—there are smooth muscles in the blood vessels of the body. What if interleukins, messengers that communicate inflammation in the body, played a role in the relaxation or failure to relax the smooth muscles in the blood vessels? So I plugged this concept into the theory, and suddenly the entire picture fit together. Furthermore, something else stood out. Everything involved in the development of heart disease was produced by the liver, an immunologic organ. Next to the skin, the liver is the largest organ in your body, but no one had ever thought of the liver being so connected to heart disease. No one except the acupuncturists and ancient Chinese healers. So now it all fit! There was an explanation behind all the factors that cause heart disease, as well as an explanation for acupuncture and the meridians used in ancient Chinese health practices. As my mentor, Professor Gordon Harrington, once pointed out, there are no new ideas, only new discoveries of old ideas and the putting together of old ideas to form a better understanding.

Now the task would be to convince other people that we were looking too narrowly at the problem and we were missing the forest for the trees, while at the same time trying to determine what we needed to do to correct all of these underlying causes. If we looked at all of the things that could go wrong and treated them, would it improve our results? I had already been focusing on dietary and lifestyle changes and had been ridiculed several times by people who didn't want to hear anything about this new approach. Later, most of my early research was presented in England, Europe, the Mediterranean region, and Japan. Interestingly enough, interleukins are now considered to be a real cause of heart disease, and inflammation is being discussed more and more. But, as with earlier findings, no one wanted to admit that pieces of the puzzle were provided by other scientists. The failure to look at other people's work and acknowledge it would continue to limit our treatment of heart disease.

Deciding to ignore the criticism and focus on my theory, which credits many other people with their contributions (I did not reinvent the wheel, and there are more than 440 references in this book), I began treating people for all the factors discussed in this book. Slowly but surely the pieces fell into place, and I developed a regimen not only for treating heart disease but for diagnosing it even in its earliest stages, where great potential exists for preventing and curing heart disease. As Galileo said, the truth is easy to understand once it is discovered. It is my hope that *Stop Inflammation Now!* will allow you to discover the truth to help you gain or regain control of your health.

Stop Inflammation Now!

1

A New Understanding of Heart Disease

*

MEREDITH WAS A 56-YEAR-OLD COMMER-
cial-airline pilot who had been grounded after she'd begun suffering chest pain that was diagnosed as angina pectoris, heart disease. Her doctor placed her on medication, but her employer told her that she would be barred from flying as long as she was ill. That meant that she was out of a job.

In addition to having heart disease, Meredith was also 25 pounds over-weight. Both conditions prompted her to adopt a well-known low-fat diet, which led to a slight weight loss and brought down her cholesterol level somewhat. Unfortunately, her chest pain persisted. Soon she could not climb a flight of stairs without experiencing a stabbing pain in her heart. She was terrified of having a sudden fatal heart attack. Her doctor suggested that she consider coronary bypass surgery, the replacement of one or more of the coronary arteries, large vessels that bring blood to the heart. She did not want to have the operation, but she knew she had to do something. Eventually she came to me.

I am a cardiologist, an internist, and the director of the Camelot Foundation in Omaha, Nebraska. I have been treating people with heart disease, as well as virtually every other type of illness, for more than two decades. Several years ago I realized that, despite remarkable advances in the diagnosis and treatment of many diseases, doctors were having far less success against heart disease than should be expected. In most cases the best that could be hoped for was that the illness could be slowed by drugs and surgery. Even then, the disease usually progressed until a fatal heart attack occurred.

Heart disease has long been understood as being caused by a handful of risk factors, some of the most important being high blood cholesterol levels, high blood pressure, overweight, and smoking. These lifestyle factors were thought to create conditions for the development of cholesterol plaques, cholesterol-filled boils, inside the coronary arteries. Doctors believed that those plaques grew until they became so large that they blocked blood flow to the heart and caused a heart attack. Although numerous risk factors were taken into account, high blood cholesterol was considered the key. When blood cholesterol went up, the theory went, cholesterol plaques were formed and the illness emerged. When it went down, the plaques receded and the illness was reversed. That, essentially, was the vision of cholesterol-caused heart disease.

Many of the facts and statistics associated with heart disease seemed to contradict this view. For example, nearly half the people who suffer heart attacks each year have what doctors describe as "normal" cholesterol levels, according to the National Heart, Lung, and Blood Institute (NHLBI). Many who died from heart attacks were later discovered on autopsy to have only small cholesterol plaques in their coronary arteries, NHLBI scientists point out. And people with heart disease who took cholesterol-lowering drugs, or lowered the fat content of their diets in order to lower their cholesterol levels, continued to suffer significant heart disease, and most died of heart attacks. Dr. Tim Church, the medical director of the Cooper Institute, a research and education center in Dallas, Texas, summed it up nicely: "The traditional risk factors—family history, diabetes, smoking, hypertension, and cholesterol—explain less than half of the cases of heart disease."

Obviously, something was wrong with our theoretical model for heart disease. Not only did some of our basic assumptions appear to be inaccurate, but treatment was not having the desired effect. I speculated that perhaps we didn't fully understand this disease; perhaps pieces of the puzzle were missing.

In 1996, I realized that one of the biggest missing puzzle pieces was the human immune system. Up until very recently, we thought that high levels of blood cholesterol were almost solely responsible for these plaques inside the arteries. What was really taking place, however, was that, as we eat foods rich in fat, protein, and calories, the levels of certain substances in the blood become elevated. Among the most important of these are a type of cholesterol known as LDL (low-density lipoprotein) cholesterol; an amino acid called homocysteine; and blood fats known as triglycerides. Triglycerides are important because they increase the level of LDL cholesterol in the blood.

LDL cholesterol and homocysteine appear in the blood as tiny spheres that are able to enter the walls of arteries. When their levels are elevated, hordes of these tiny balls infiltrate the artery wall. Once there, they oxidize, or decay. The immune system recognizes these decaying fragments as a threat to health and immediately sends immune cells into the artery tissue to gobble up these decaying LDL and homocysteine particles.

When the immune cells consume the decaying particles of LDL cholesterol and homocysteine, they become bloated. These bloated immune cells combine to form a yellow growth, also known as a "fatty streak," inside the artery wall. As more LDL and homocysteine particles appear, more immune cells gobble up the decaying balls, causing the streak to become bigger. Soon it grows so large that it causes the artery tissue to harden; eventually it forms a kind of boil, filled with cholesterol and the debris from immune cells and other blood constituents, that protrudes out into the artery passageway. The presence of these plaques inside the arteries is called atherosclerosis.

As more LDL cholesterol and homocysteine pour into the blood, more immune cells enter the artery tissue, in an attempt to clean away these decaying particles. The net effect is that the plaques grow even larger.

Something else takes place that is especially dangerous: immune cells make the plaques unstable and more likely to erupt, much like a volcano. They force the plaque to grow bigger from within. But immune cells also produce a substance that wears away the covering that caps the boil. These two actions—enlarging the boil and wearing away the covering—increase the likelihood of the boil's erupting.

Once the plaque blows, it spews forth its contents of cholesterol and cellular debris and leaves an open wound in the artery wall. Whenever the body recognizes a wound, it forms a blood clot, or a scab, over the wound's opening. That covering, known as a thrombus, can become so large that it can block blood from flowing to the heart or brain and thus cause a heart attack or stroke. Or it can break free from the plaque, float downstream, and get caught in a narrow passage within the artery, where it can block blood flow to the heart or brain and have the same effect.

All of this begins with having excess LDL cholesterol and high levels of triglycerides and homocysteine in your bloodstream. Homocysteine and other substances also promote the body's tendency to form larger clots, which makes the thrombus even more deadly. The immune reaction that helps create these events is referred to as inflammation.

Inflammation is caused when the immune system sends out immune cells to fight an infection or excess quantities of toxins in the blood, including excess cholesterol. Whenever immune cells attack a bacteria, virus, or high levels of toxins, it creates an array of side effects that we typically associate with inflammation, including heat, redness, and swelling. Those same characteristics are occurring inside the artery wall, causing the artery to become deformed, swollen, and bulbous with erupting plaques. Inflammation, I now realized, was the root cause of heart attacks and strokes.

LDL cholesterol, triglycerides, and homocysteine are not the only culprits triggering this inflammatory reaction within the arteries. After further study, I found that there are at least 12 conditions that set off the destructive inflammatory response. This new information explained why heart disease is not being treated successfully today. Doctors are only dealing with a handful of the risk factors that cause the illness. If your cholesterol level is normal, your doctor may believe that you are free of heart disease, when in fact you may have significant heart disease and might even be on the brink of a heart attack. This explains why so many people with normal cholesterol levels have heart attacks and strokes—because the illness is caused by more than just high LDL cholesterol levels.

It also explains other apparent anomalies in the heart disease picture. In the past, small plaques were not viewed as particularly dangerous, but later we learned that small plaques cause most heart attacks. How could this be? The answer was inflammation, which makes even small plaques highly unstable, more likely to rupture than large ones, and more likely to form large blood clots that could kill.

Unless all 12 risk factors are treated effectively, heart disease cannot be brought under control, but fortunately all 12 risk factors can be reduced to their healthy ranges. On the basis of the new data, I designed a treatment program for controlling inflammation and reversing heart disease. I used this approach to treat Meredith.

First I ran a series of blood tests and found that her blood cholesterol level was 220 milligrams per deciliter of blood. An ideal blood cholesterol level is 150 mg/dL or lower. Her blood fat, or triglyceride, level was 200 mg/dL. As with cholesterol, the ideal triglyceride level is less than 150 mg/dL. Other tests showed that Meredith's homocysteine level was 12.6 µmol/L; a normal level for women is less than 10. She also had those 20-plus pounds to lose, which contributed to her heart condition by forcing her heart to work harder.

"So, my cholesterol is too high, right?" Meredith said to me, after I got her blood tests back.

"Yes," I said, "but that's only one of your problems. Heart disease is caused by a dozen factors, not just cholesterol. All of them have to be restored to healthy ranges if we are to cure you of heart disease."

I explained that the underlying process that leads to heart attacks is inflammation. "Think of inflammation as the result of having all these toxic waste substances dumped into your artery tissue. Your immune cells try to clean up the mess, but in the process they create swelling, heat, and redness, resulting in highly volatile boils that are prone to erupting. When they rupture, they release their contents into the blood and leave a wound in the artery. The body forms a scab over the wound, but the scab can be so large that it can block blood flow to your heart and cause a heart attack."

"It's like when the pus in a boil bursts out and the body tries to heal it, right?" Meredith said.

"That's right," I said. "Only, in your arteries, the healing process—the formation of a scab—is extremely dangerous."

"What causes inflammation?" Meredith asked.

"Lots of things," I said. "In the case of heart disease, many of the foods we eat. Also, overweight, lack of exercise, smoking, and high levels of certain chemicals in the blood."

"Which foods cause inflammation?" she asked.

"Well, a lot of foods that we typically think of as bad for the heart because of their fat content, such as red meat, dairy products, eggs, and fried foods," I said. "They all trigger inflammation. But many other foods that contain little or no fat and no cholesterol do it, too—foods that we used to think of as safe, such as low-fat muffins, bagels, white bread, and pastries—any food that is processed or contains lots of simple sugars. In fact, diets that are rich in calories—even when they are low in fat—can cause inflammation and heart disease."

"If cholesterol isn't the answer, then what is?" Meredith asked.

"We have to reduce the inflammation that's occurring throughout your body," I said. "As the inflammation cools, the cholesterol plaques shrink, and the arteries that lead to your heart, brain, and other organs will open. At that point, you're going to feel like a new person."

"How can we do that?" she asked.

"We do it in a two-phase process," I said. "Phase 1 requires some pretty serious changes in your diet and the inclusion of some supplements. Think of Phase 1 as a kind of temporary cleansing of your body. You won't be fasting—you'll be eating foods that you can enjoy and take pleasure from. But these foods will cause a rapid transformation in your health. You'll lose weight quickly. Your cholesterol, triglyceride, and homocysteine levels will fall rapidly into healthy ranges. Your heart will get stronger, as will your immune system. And you'll feel great. You'll have a lot more energy. Your body will feel lighter and healthier and more alive. You'll look many years younger. But it will require some discipline. Once we achieve our goals for Phase 1, you'll move on to Phase 2 of the program, which includes a wider diet, a little more exercise, and some supplements."

"I want to do it," Meredith said. "I'm ready to change my life and get back into the pilot's seat."

Overview of the Fleming Program

During Phase 1 of the Fleming Program, you eat just vegetables, legumes, and fruits. There is a wide array of vegetables on the program, everything from sweet potatoes and squash to onions, carrots, and mushrooms. Also on the diet are fruits, and lots of them: apples, oranges, cherries, peaches, bananas, and dark grapes. There is a strong emphasis on foods and condiments that strengthen immune function and at the same time reduce inflammation. We need to strengthen the immune system because, for many of us, it has been forced to overwork for most of our lives. Unfortunately, the standard American diet does not supply the nutrients the immune system needs to be strong. Forcing the immune system to overwork while failing to give it what it needs makes us vulnerable to a whole range of illnesses, including heart disease, cancer, and many infectious diseases.

We want to take the stress off the immune system while we make it stronger. The Fleming Program Phase 1 diet can do both. It's rich in immune boosters as well as foods that reduce inflammation, such as blueberries, flax seeds, and cruciferous vegetables (in the family Cruciferae) such as broccoli, cabbage, cauliflower, collard greens, kale, and mustard greens.

Phase 1 also includes a supplement regimen of folic acid (part of the B complex), vitamins B_6 and B_{12}, and an antioxidant formula. These vitamins lower homocysteine levels and reduce free radicals, which are highly destructive oxygen molecules that damage artery tissue and promote atherosclerosis, the formation of cholesterol plaques. Finally, there is a Phase 1 exercise regimen, which consists primarily of walking.

Meredith made immediate progress on Phase 1. It wasn't long before she experienced the kind of transformation that I had outlined to her at the outset of our work together. Four months after her initial visit with me, Meredith's blood cholesterol level had dropped to 140 mg/dL, her triglycerides were 130 mg/dL, and her homocysteine was 8 µmol/L. She had lost 25 pounds. Her chest pain was completely gone. She was off all medication, and her electrocardiogram showed no sign of heart disease. Best of all, she was flying again. Once she had achieved the Phase 1 goals, I placed her on Phase 2 of the program, which includes a more liberal diet, an array of anti-inflammatory foods and supplements, and a Phase 2 exercise program.

How was all of this possible? We did it by controlling the 12 risk factors that bring about inflammatory immune response and by drastically reducing the causes of inflammation in her body. From there, we let nature take its course.

The 12 Links in a Chain Reaction

Below is a brief summary of the 12 essential risk factors in the inflammatory reaction that creates heart disease. The program that you are about to begin can restore each of these 12 factors to healthy ranges and in the process restore your health.

1. Cholesterol

Cholesterol appears in your arteries as tiny fatlike balls of lipoproteins. As mentioned earlier, one type of cholesterol, low-density cholesterol, causes heart disease. The particles of another type of cholesterol, HDL (high-density lipoproteins), attach themselves to the LDL particles and transport them to the liver. Thus, HDL is considered "good cholesterol," because it protects you from heart disease, and LDL is termed "bad cholesterol," because it causes the illness.

Blood cholesterol—specifically, LDL cholesterol—is the first link in the 12-part chain. Cholesterol buildup triggers the immune reaction that can lead to a heart attack or a stroke. Therefore, the first thing we must do is to bring down the LDL cholesterol level. LDL cholesterol is found in saturated fats. Phase 1 of my program eliminates all saturated fat, so that your cholesterol levels will fall quickly to normal levels. Phase 2 allows some saturated fat, but it is well within healthy limits and therefore will maintain your LDL blood cholesterol at a safe level.

2. Triglycerides

Triglycerides are tiny globules of fat in your blood. Triglyceride levels become elevated when you consume excess amounts of saturated fats, or the fats that are typically found in animal foods. Triglyceride levels also go up when you consume excess amounts of calories, processed foods, and processed sugars. In fact, triglyceride levels can become so high that they turn the blood thick and white from the overwhelming amount of fat in it. Saturated fats are those that are unable to receive additional hydrogen (hydrogenated) atoms and tend to be solid at room temperature. They usually come from animal sources and processed foods. In a great many cases, a person who has high triglycerides is also overweight. He or she may already have adult-onset (type 2) diabetes, or may be at high risk for developing it. This combination of high triglycerides, overweight, and diabetes dramatically increases the chances of having a heart attack. It also gives rise to an array of other problems, including chest pain (angina pectoris) from insufficient blood flow to the heart; claudication (insufficient blood flow to the legs); and elevated insulin (high levels of the hormone produced by the body to make blood sugar available to cells). High insulin, as we will see in detail in chapter 3, causes weight gain and leads to an array of serious illnesses. This constellation of symptoms—excess weight, high insulin, and high triglycerides—is also often associated with liver and digestive disorders, chronic fatigue, and high blood pressure. Most people who suffer from this syndrome feel lousy.

Phase 1 of the Fleming Program brings triglyceride levels down quickly. Since approximately 20 percent of triglycerides are converted to LDL cholesterol, the lowering of triglycerides also lowers LDL blood cholesterol levels.

3. Excess Weight

The foods that trigger an inflammatory reaction and create heart disease also cause weight gain. Excess body weight is associated with an array of other disorders that cause inflammation, such as high cholesterol levels, high triglycerides, imbalanced hormones, low-fiber diet, and lack of exercise. This is one of the reasons why it is a major risk factor in heart attack, stroke, diabetes, and cancer.

No program for treating or preventing heart disease, or any other major illness, can be successful unless it is also highly effective at causing weight loss. And Phase 1 is the best and healthiest way that I am familiar with to lose weight.

4. Homocysteine

One of the key events that touches off an inflammatory reaction is the creation of a wound in the artery wall. Another is the formation of a large blood clot over that wound. Homocysteine contributes to both events.

Homocysteine is an amino acid whose blood levels become elevated as a result of excess consumption of red meat and other animal-protein sources. In order to metabolize animal proteins, your body utilizes folic acid and vitamins B_6 and B_{12}. If heavy meat consumption lowers your body's levels of these vitamins, your homocysteine levels will increase to dangerously high levels. These protective vitamins are found in plant foods, such as green vegetables and beans. People on high-protein diets, of course, eat lots of protein but are told to eat lower levels of plant foods.

Elevated homocysteine acts like burning acid on your artery walls, creating injuries throughout the arterial system. Once the artery is wounded, hordes of immune cells descend on the site of the injury, making the vessel highly inflamed. At the same time, homocysteine increases the blood's tendency to form clots. In combination, wounding the vessel and making the blood more likely to clot are two important steps in the creation of a thrombus and a heart attack.

Phase 1 of the Fleming Program dramatically reduces homocysteine levels to optimal ranges.

5. Antioxidants

LDL cholesterol particles oxidize and break down—they decay—when they come in contact with highly reactive oxygen molecules known as oxidants. This decay causes the immune system to spring into action, and thus begins the plaque-formation process. Oxidation, therefore, is a pivotal event in the creation of both inflammation and the formation of plaques.

Oxidation breaks down and deforms cells, causing tissue to shrink, wrinkle, and age. Oxidants cause scars to form in organs such as the liver and the intestinal tract. Oxidation is the underlying cause of most of the illnesses we suffer from today, including heart disease, high blood pressure, cataracts, and Alzheimer's and Parkinson's diseases. Oxidants also deform DNA and cause some cells to become malignant.

To a great extent the level of oxidants in our bloodstream and tissues is determined by the foods we eat, whether or not we smoke, the extent of our exposure to the sun's ultraviolet rays, and the toxins we encounter from the environment. Dietary fat is a principal source of oxidants, as are alcohol, processed foods, and pesticides.

The antidote to oxidation is antioxidants, substances that counteract oxidants and bring a halt to the oxidation process. The primary source of antioxidants is plant foods: vegetables, grains, beans, and fruit. The antioxidants in these foods slow and even stop the oxidation process and thus prevent plaque formation. Antioxidants also boost the immune system and the body's other cancer-fighting forces. Phases 1 and 2 of my program are rich in antioxidants.

6. Exercise

Moderate exercise lowers levels of insulin, triglycerides, estrogen, and fibrinogen (see next section). All of these are pro-inflammatory substances, which is why moderate exercise reduces inflammation throughout the body. Moderate exercise also reduces weight, promotes the elimination of waste products from the body, and boosts immune function. It strengthens the heart, promotes better circulation, and reduces the risk of cancer. Exercise is an essential part of any health program. All of these benefits and many more can be experienced by doing the gentle exercise program described in chapter 4. The program is safe, effective, and easy to maintain.

7. Fibrinogen

Fibrinogen is a protein that increases the blood's tendency to form clots. Many factors increase production of fibrinogen, including diets rich in fat and animal proteins. As fibrinogen levels go up, the blood forms more clots, which means the risk of heart attack increases significantly.

Following the Fleming Program brings fibrinogen levels into safe ranges, thus reducing the blood's tendency to form dangerous clots and greatly reducing the risk of heart attack.

8. Growth Factors

Growth factors are substances that promote cellular growth. They regulate the behavior of arteries, causing them to expand and contract, elevate fibrinogen levels, cause cells to multiply, and trigger inflammatory reactions. For all of these reasons, you want to have balanced growth factors in your bloodstream. Unfortunately, growth factors become elevated when we eat diets rich in red meat, dairy products, poultry, and eggs. A diet based on plant foods dramatically lowers growth factors and promotes the opening of blood vessels, including the coronary arteries.

Growth-factor levels drop quickly into the safe ranges on my program.

9. Cytokines and Leukotrienes

Whenever the cells of your immune system spring into action, they have to communicate with each other in order to coordinate their attack on a disease-causing agent or cancer cell. Cytokines and leukotrienes, chemicals that are part of the immune system, make that communication possible. In addition to communication, these chemicals stimulate actions by immune cells. Leukotrienes can cause a wide variety of reactions in your system, including inflammation and constriction of blood vessels and arteries. They can also promote atherosclerosis.

Phase 1 of the Fleming Program brings cytokines and leukotrienes into balance and Phase 2 keeps them there, thus cooling the inflammatory response, opening arteries, and maximizing blood flow to the heart, brain, and other organs.

10. Complement

Complement is a protein produced by the immune system. It roams the blood, seeking out bacteria that pose a threat to health. Once complement recognizes the presence of a pathogen, it attaches itself to the bacterium and pokes holes in its cell membrane, thus killing the organism. Sometimes, however, complement is a bit indiscriminate in its hole-punching activities, attacking not only bacteria but also large and small arteries, thus releasing blood into the tissues. Frequently, the redness that you see around a cut is blood that has been released from vessels after complement has poked a few too many holes in the nearby blood vessels. In fact, complement may deliberately punch holes in arteries to bring an even greater immune response to the area, thus ensuring that whatever threat to health may be present will be destroyed by the overwhelming reaction from the immune system.

The more inflammation there is in any part of the body, the more complement is attracted there. The more complement, the more holes are poked into artery walls. The more holes, the more inflammation. Hence, the vicious cycle.

On Phase 1 of the program, inflammation drops dramatically, and complement levels fall into balance. Phase 2 keeps both the inflammation and the complement levels down.

11. Bacteria

One of the most surprising discoveries recently made in heart disease research has been that cholesterol plaque is rife with bacteria. The bigger the plaque, the more bacteria live within it. Bacteria are to the immune system what a red cape is to a bull. The immune cells arrive like a herd of bulls, and pretty soon the place is a mass of inflammation that fuels the growth of a cholesterol plaque. Also the presence of highly active immune cells, coupled with an abundance of LDL cholesterol, makes the plaque increasingly unstable and more likely to rupture. With each rupture, the clot grows larger and the chances of a heart attack grow even greater.

One of the ways I treat heart disease today is by reducing the presence of bacteria in the system with a mild antibiotic. (All the information you need to share with your doctor is in chapter 7.)

12. Protect Your Arteries

Any injury to the artery wall triggers an immune or inflammatory reaction within the artery. Most of those injuries come from levels of LDL cholesterol, homocysteine, and complement, but some come from medical procedures themselves. Invasive diagnostic tests and procedures such as angiography and coronary balloon angioplasty can actually promote the growth of the illness. In chapter 8, I provide a guide to appropriate medical care and help you and your doctor determine when such procedures are appropriate and when they should be avoided.

The Fire in Your Arteries

Each of these 12 risk factors influences in its own way how your immune system functions, thus determining the extent of the inflammation in your body. The key to ridding ourselves of heart disease is to keep the immune system healthy and inflammation low.

The word "inflammation" originated with the Greeks and was used to indicate a fire within the body. That is still a highly accurate description, for the symptoms of inflammation include heat, redness, fever, pain, rash, and swelling. In short, a fire within.

The immune system is composed primarily of many different types of white blood cells and proteins. Some of those proteins act directly to destroy viruses and bacteria, while others serve as messengers, sending information back and forth between immune cells and white blood cells. The immune system is essentially an awesome army that is on active duty every day of your life. It has the power to destroy just about anything that threatens your health and life. Under healthy, normal conditions, the army is quiet. Oh, there are skirmishes here and there—a small infection in a cut that must be contained, for example, or a bacterium or virus that has been ingested and must be destroyed before it spreads. Every day, you produce hundreds of potentially cancerous cells, and the immune system recognizes them and destroys them before they destroy you. That's normal, everyday business for your immune system. Whenever the immune system takes on a disease-causing agent, it launches an incredibly varied and creative response that we refer to today as inflammation.

Inflammation, as I have said, is essential to our survival. But the more disease-causing agents you have in your system, the more inflammation you have throughout your body. When inflammation becomes excessive, your chances of heart disease increase dramatically.

As it turns out, researchers have discovered that inflammation is a factor in most of the dangerous diseases we face—illnesses such as diabetes, most forms of cancer, high blood pressure, arthritis, asthma, glaucoma, and Alzheimer's and Parkinson's diseases. The 12 risk factors that I have identified are the primary causes of inflammation. As I will show in this book, by reducing inflammation, the Fleming Program can help prevent—and in many cases treat—most of the major illnesses we suffer from today.

This book focuses primarily on heart disease, but the Fleming Program can also be highly effective at helping your body fight malignant cells and tumors. It can therefore be an important adjunct treatment for people with cancer. I have included a self-help program for people with cancer, diabetes, and other serious illnesses.

Apart from their role in the creation of major illness, the 12 risk factors also directly affect how we feel each day and determine how rapidly we age. They promote weight gain; cause the loss of energy and endurance; reduce our mental acuity and promote memory loss; lower mood; and increase anxiety. As these 12 risk factors get out of control, we experience the inexplicable dread that arises when we know that we're getting weaker and losing control of our lives.

On the other hand, when these 12 factors are brought into safe ranges, you can restore your heart to normal, vigorous function; lower your elevated blood pressure; enjoy significant and healthful weight loss; and experience a dramatic improvement in energy, mental clarity, and memory. You can protect yourself from major illnesses. You will very likely feel a strong sense of well-being and elevated mood. In short, this program can transform your life.

C-RP: An Essential Test

A doctor can determine the amount of inflammation occurring in your body with a simple blood test that measures a protein known as C-reactive protein (C-RP), which is produced by the liver and rises within 24 hours of an increase in the inflammation in your body. We now know that elevated C-RP levels are highly accurate predictors of cardiovascular health or illness, especially when they are combined with blood cholesterol results. In fact, we can use these two tests to accurately predict the likelihood of your having a heart attack because, as shown above, the more inflammation in your arteries, the more unstable your cholesterol plaques. Unstable plaques that erupt and cause a blood clot are the primary cause of heart attack and stroke.

A C-RP test is at least as important as a blood cholesterol test, and some researchers say that it's more important, because some studies have shown that it may be a more accurate predictor of heart attack. A study published in *The New England Journal of Medicine* (Ridker 2002) found that women who had high C-reactive protein levels were twice as likely to have a heart attack or stroke as women with high cholesterol levels. Researchers from Harvard University followed 27,939 women at Brigham and Women's Hospital in Boston for eight years. They found that there was a higher statistical correlation between high C-RP levels than with high LDL cholesterol levels.

The irony here is that the immune system's ability to fight back with inflammation is one of the reasons humans have survived for 2 million years. The immune system triggers inflammatory responses in order to destroy disease-causing bacteria and viruses. You wouldn't want to take away that defensive protection, not unless you wanted to live inside a sterile bubble all your life. Yet inflammation is exactly what destroys our arteries and leads to heart attacks and strokes. How, you might ask, does a normal, healthy reaction become an out-of-control fire inside our arteries? The answer is that by overworking our immune systems with our diets and lifestyles we start the fire that eventually kills us.

Heart Disease: Everyone's Problem

Sooner or later, heart disease concerns us all. No one is immune. Either you're doing something to protect your heart and arteries or you're very likely on the road to a heart attack or a stroke. According to the American Heart Association (AHA), heart disease will kill about half of all Americans, and this year, more than 1 million Americans will experience a heart attack. Of those who survive the first one, nearly two thirds will have another one. Fifty million U.S. citizens have high blood pressure, one of the primary risk factors for heart attack and stroke. Once you have been diagnosed with heart disease, your chances of dying suddenly are five to seven times that of the general population.

Heart disease is the leading killer of men and women worldwide. Contrary to widely held misconceptions, more women than men die from cardiovascular disease each year—more than 500,000.

These statistics all point to an undeniable conclusion: Despite all the advances medical science has made in the diagnosis and treatment of this disease, there is still no sure medical cure for this illness. Even when you lower the fat content of your diet, or when you combine a low-fat diet with cholesterol-lowering drugs, your chances of making a full recovery are highly unpredictable—in fact, you may even get worse.

Nowhere is this more painfully illustrated than in the case of U.S. Vice President Richard Cheney. The vice president suffered his first heart attack in 1978, at the age of 37. Throughout the past 25 years, Cheney has received state-of-the-art health care. Yet he has had three more heart attacks since. In 1988 he underwent quadruple bypass surgery. In 2000 he had a small tube, called a stent, inserted into one of his coronary arteries in an attempt to keep the vessel open, but by the following March cholesterol plaques had penetrated the tube and closed the artery by 90 percent. As a consequence, he underwent balloon angioplasty, a procedure that involves threading a catheter tube into the coronary arteries and inflating a balloon that crushes the cholesterol plaques against the artery wall, thus forcibly opening the artery. In addition to all of this, Cheney has received all of the available medications, including cholesterol-lowering drugs. Yet his condition throughout the past two-and-a-half decades has remained perilous, and he was hospitalized again in March 2001 for chest pain.

Since September 11, 2001, the vice president has remained largely out of the public eye, except for an occasional appearance to reassure us of his presence on the job. But before his retreat from visibility, the nation held its collective breath as we watched him go through his very demanding schedule. Many cardiologists quietly speculated that the vice president might not survive his four years in office.

There are at least three reasons why the current medical treatments are not having the desired effects.

1. Medical Treatments Are Inadequate to Cure the Illness

There is no cure for heart disease in the medical arsenal. Drug treatment, as necessary as it often is, generally provides only short-term, palliative relief.

Drugs cannot and do not treat all the risk factors that combine to create inflammation and heart disease. Even the medications that lower blood cholesterol cannot lower it sufficiently to reverse the illness. These two facts explain why the illness often progresses even while a patient is under a doctor's care.

As for surgery, that, too, provides only temporary relief. Bypass surgery, which replaces one or more of the a coronary arteries, can restore blood flow to the heart. Unfortunately, the new vessels become blocked, or occluded, just as the old ones did. Studies show that 8 to 12 percent of all bypasses close significantly even before a patient leaves the hospital. A year after the surgery, 12 to 20 percent of the bypassed arteries have closed. Five years later, more than 25 percent are closed, and after 15 years, 85 percent of them are blocked again.

The other common procedure, angioplasty, has even poorer long-term results. Within six months of the procedure, 25 to 50 percent of the vessels are blocked and in need of more surgery. These facts explain why the vice president's illness has steadily progressed. Thus, so far nothing his doctors have been able to do for him has truly taken him out of danger.

After extensively investigating the Cheney experience, in May 2001 *The Magazine*, the magazine for the American Association of Retired People (AARP), stated, in an article titled "Heart disease: a lot is up to you. Cheney case suggests high-tech science isn't enough," that "the real lesson of Cheney's case, top cardiologists say, is that high-tech medical intervention, valuable as it is, is no substitute for lifestyle changes."

2. Too Little Emphasis on the Importance of Diet and Lifestyle Change

The second reason that more people are not being cured is because doctors often fail to tell their patients the limitations of medical treatment. In too many cases, the patient is led to believe that drugs or surgery (or both) represent a cure. After undergoing surgery in which five of his coronary arteries were replaced, the famed Chicago Bears linebacker Dick Butkus was asked by an ESPN reporter how he felt. Butkus said that he felt great after the operation and could now go back to drinking beer and eating steak. Butkus may well have been joking, but he nonetheless communicated what many people believe. Unfortunately, surgery alone is no cure, as the vice president and numerous others have so painfully discovered.

The simple, inescapable truth is that the typical Western diet is the cause of inflammatory heart disease, just as appropriate dietary change is the cure. If doctors explained to patients that there is only so much that medicine can do, they would force patients to take responsibility for doing their part in the treatment process. This would be harsh medicine at first, but it would be honest and realistic, and ultimately it would save thousands of lives.

3. Most Forms of Dietary Change Are Inadequate

Appropriate diet, used alone or in combination with drug treatment, is the only way to shrink the cholesterol plaques and cure coronary heart disease. The healing process is greatly enhanced when diet is combined with exercise. So which diet and what type of change will bring about the desired results? That's not as easy to answer as you might think, despite all the publicity that has been lavished on certain very popular dietary programs.

In 1994 I conducted a study in which I carefully examined the results of a well-known very low-fat and low-cholesterol diet and yoga program for 39 people with proven heart disease. All the people in the study adhered closely to the diet and yoga program for one year. They also received drug treatment to further lower their blood cholesterol levels.

I examined the results of each person's before-and-after PET (positron emission tomography) scans, a highly accurate test for determining the extent of atherosclerosis in the coronary arteries. One third of the patients got better on the program, meaning that the plaques in their coronary arteries shrank. One third experienced no change in their condition, and one third got worse, meaning their plaques got bigger.

How was this possible? Here was a program that dramatically lowered fat and cholesterol in the diet. The program provided people with cholesterol-lowering drugs, and the regular yoga exercises presumably lowered stress. Still, the results were less than impressive. In fact, my study showed that the results of this program were highly unpredictable. If a low-fat, low-cholesterol diet was the answer to heart disease, why didn't everyone get better? We were missing something, but what was it? I wondered.

I searched the medical literature for risk factors that might be involved in the genesis of atherosclerosis but were going unnoticed or underappreciated to that point. I soon discovered numerous scientific studies that pointed to an as yet unrecognized player in the creation of cholesterol plaques. That player was the immune system.

The Fleming Program

Have you ever watched someone perform a sport with real gusto, or looked with true appreciation as someone effortlessly ran past you, and then thought to yourself, I would love to get back into shape? Or have you been overweight and longed to be at your natural healthy weight again? Have you ever yearned to have your body working really well; to enjoy deep and restful sleep; to wake up refreshed and full of energy; to go through the day at full tilt? Have you had the following thought: I would love to do something that would drain my body of all the poisons I've been carrying around for years and make my system clean again?

The Fleming Program offers you that opportunity. You can make your heart strong again; rid yourself of excess weight; cleanse your body of toxins that fill your tissues and fluids; let your organs fully breathe; and experience what it is like to be healthy and fully alive. I believe that these goals are worth making a sustained effort to achieve.

As you now know, the Fleming Program is made up of two phases. Phase 1 is powerful short-term "medicine," based on a diet made up exclusively of vegetables and fruit. People who adopt this diet say that after a short adjustment period, they have no trouble remaining on the regimen. In fact, I have patients who, long after they are able to go on to Phase 2, remain largely on Phase 1 for the simple reason that they enjoy eating this way, and because it gives them tremendous energy and keeps their weight down.

The Phase 1 diet brings all 12 risk factors into the balanced, healthy ranges and drastically reduces your chances of suffering a heart attack or stroke. It also brings about rapid and healthful weight loss.

Phase 2 is highly flexible. It gives you the means to maintain the benefits you have derived from Phase 1 but also gives you much greater freedom in your food choices. During Phase 2, you are allowed to eat certain amounts of animal foods and certain oils, such as olive oil. You will have no trouble sustaining Phase 2, no matter what your lifestyle is. You can travel, eat in restaurants, and enjoy your life to the fullest.

Both phases have four simple parts:

1. Avoid foods that promote inflammation.
2. Include foods that reduce inflammation.

3. Take supplements that reduce inflammation.
4. Exercise to reduce inflammation.

1. Avoid Pro-inflammatory Foods

The foods that promote inflammation and should be avoided are the following:

- Foods that contain saturated fats. These include red meat, dairy products, poultry, eggs, and fish. You should also avoid coconut oil and palm kernel oil. During Phase 1, I urge you to avoid all of these foods, at least until the Phase 1 goals are met for weight, cholesterol, homocysteine, fibrinogen, and other risk factors (described in chapter 9). Limited amounts of these foods are permitted in Phase 2 (described in chapter 10).
- Foods that contain omega-6 polyunsaturated fats, specifically vegetable oils, such as corn oil, safflower oil, and sunflower oil.
- Foods that contain trans-fatty acids, such as margarine, processed foods, pastries, doughnuts, and many baked flour products.
- Dairy foods, including cow's milk, cheese, and yogurt. These foods are highly inflammatory and promote the production of inflammatory cytokines, including insulin-like growth factor 1 (IGF-1). IGF-1 is related not only to inflammation but also to many forms of cancer, including breast and prostate cancers. In Phase 2 you can reintroduce some dairy products into your diet—if you desire dairy foods—without causing excessive inflammatory reactions.
- All foods that contain refined sugar.
- All processed foods, which are rich in calories and consequently promote inflammation. These include all breads, rolls, muffins, cookies, cakes, chips, and soft drinks.

2. Include Anti-inflammatory Foods

While eliminating the pro-inflammatory foods, you will include foods that are anti-inflammatory:

- A wide assortment of vegetables. In general, plant-based diets are anti-inflammatory and boost the immune system.

- Cruciferous vegetables, such as broccoli, cabbage, cauliflower, collard greens, kale, mustard greens, and Brussels sprouts. All are highly anti-inflammatory.
- Vegetables in the allium family, including garlic, onions, and scallions. Very anti-inflammatory.
- Flaxseeds and pumpkin seeds.
- Selected fruits, including blueberries, grapes, plums, and citrus fruits.
- Foods rich in vitamin C, especially broccoli, leafy green vegetables, and citrus fruits.
- Foods that contain vitamin E, including whole grains, almonds, and some seeds.
- Foods rich in selenium, including walnuts, Brazil nuts, and seafood.
- High-fiber foods. In general, fibrous foods—whole grains, vegetables, and fruits—lower inflammation by binding with pro-inflammatory substances and eliminating them from your system.

3. Take Supplements

You should also take certain food-based, anti-inflammatory supplements:

- A daily vitamin and mineral supplement that includes vitamins B_6 and B_{12} and folic acid.
- A daily antioxidant formula.

4. Exercise

In Phase 1, the exercise is daily walking. In Phase 2, the exercise can include stretching, yoga, walking, and some gentle, noncompetitive games.

In the chapters that follow, I will describe how each of the 12 risk factors can be brought into balance and restored to healthy ranges. I will show you how heart disease and other serious illnesses arise, and how they can be successfully defeated. A lifetime of good health awaits you if you are willing to read on and to adopt the program that can change your life.

Cholesterol and Triglycerides

IN AUGUST 2000, KAREN CAME TO SEE me with chronic chest pain that I soon discovered was caused by coronary heart disease. She had a cholesterol level of 215 mg/dL, triglycerides of 202 mg/dL, and a C-reactive protein (C-RP) level of 1.9 mg/dL. C-RP should not be higher than 0.5 mg/dL, and Karen's was way above that. Furthermore, Karen was about 40 pounds overweight. She was only 33 years old.

Chest pain, or angina pectoris, is caused by insufficient blood flow to the heart. Like any muscle, the heart requires more blood and oxygen whenever it is forced to work harder, such as when you climb a flight of stairs, do some gardening, play a sport, or even experience stress. Cholesterol plaques can impede the flow of blood and oxygen to the heart by creating a partial obstruction in the artery, especially when demand for both goes up during exercise. That causes chest pain. But there's another way that chest pain can be caused, even before plaques start protruding into the artery pathway.

During exercise, healthy arteries expand to allow more blood flow to the heart. However, inflammation and the early stages of plaque formation within the artery wall make it hard and inflexible and prevent it from expanding normally. Consequently, when you start to exercise, and your heart demands more blood and oxygen, the artery is too hard and inflexible to expand. It cannot permit more blood to flow to the heart, which causes angina.

Karen's chest pain appeared whenever she exerted herself for about half an hour. She loved gardening and taking walks, but increasingly she found that she was unable to work in her garden or walk for any length of time without experiencing the terrifying pain, and soon the pain and fear associated with it caused her to limit her activities. That only heightened her fears of having a heart attack and dying prematurely.

Karen ate a diet rich in animal foods, including hamburgers, steak, bacon, sausage, and lots of dairy products, such as milk, cheese, and yogurt. She also ate plenty of processed foods, such as white bread, rolls, and the occasional muffin or pastry. She knew her diet was bad but didn't really know which diet to follow to help her overcome her disease. That was one of the reasons she came to me.

I told Karen that I would prescribe a drug to relieve her chest pain in the short term. "That will make you more secure and less worried about your heart," I told her, "but in order for us to actually eliminate the heart disease, we have to lower your blood cholesterol and triglyceride levels, as well as your weight. We cannot cure you of heart disease unless we do that. Ideally, we'd like to get your cholesterol, triglyceride level, and weight down fairly quickly. We want to see some real results in less than a month."

I placed Karen on the Phase 1 program, and to our mutual satisfaction she experienced a very rapid transformation. Within weeks, her cholesterol, triglycerides, C-RP levels, and weight all fell significantly. Within six months, her cholesterol level was 156 mg/dL. Her triglycerides were 112 mg/dL, and her C-RP was 0.3 mg/dL. Her weight was 121 pounds.

I also performed a single photon emission computed tomography (SPECT) test on her heart. This is a type of nuclear cardiac imaging—a procedure in which a small quantity of a radioactive substance (called an isotope) is injected into a vein in the arm of the patient, to be absorbed by the patient's heart and coronary arteries, where the radioactive substance can be seen and interpreted by equipment outside the patient's body. Different nuclear cardiac imaging techniques involve different types of cameras and different isotopes.

The most common are the planar scan, the PET (positron emission tomography) scan, and the SPECT scan. (The biggest difference between planar and SPECT techniques is that the SPECT camera can move around the patient, whereas the planar camera is fixed, and then repositioned around the patient as needed. PET scans are also fixed cameras but have detectors all the way around the person's heart.) A SPECT test can provide extremely accurate information about the condition and function of the heart and the coronary arteries. In fact, more—and more accurate—information can be obtained through nuclear imaging than from an angiogram, the standard test used to examine the coronary arteries. An angiogram can only see inside the artery pathway; it cannot see the artery tissue itself, nor can it give doctors much information about the heart muscle.

Karen's second SPECT test showed a significant increase in blood flow to her heart compared with her first SPECT test. She experienced no chest pain, even when she exerted herself well beyond her previous limits. I took her off the drug and pronounced her well.

Karen was ecstatic, to say the least. It was as if a butterfly had emerged from a large, oval chrysalis. She had more energy, clarity of mind, and dynamism than she had experienced since childhood. I continued to see her every six weeks or so for the next six months. She had no trouble keeping the weight off, and her heart disease had vanished.

High Blood Cholesterol: Where the Disease Begins

Heart disease is an inflammatory disease that occurs within the walls of the arteries. The inflammatory chain reaction that leads to cholesterol plaques and heart attacks is triggered most often by high blood cholesterol.

Imagine cholesterol as tiny, fatlike globules that float inside your blood stream. These globules, called lipids, ride on the backs of proteins, called lipoproteins. Cholesterol may be LDL, low-density lipoprotein, which creates cholesterol plaques and heart attacks, or HDL, high-density lipoprotein, which helps to protect you from heart disease by having an anti-inflammatory effect on arteries.

Strictly speaking, it's not the LDL cholesterol in your blood that's a problem but the cholesterol that gets deposited in your arteries. These tiny LDL globules are able to enter and exit the walls of your arteries, passing between the cells in the artery lining. When overall blood cholesterol becomes excessive, the LDL particles bunch up inside your artery and get stuck there. They're like too many fat men trying to get out of the same door at the same time. They can't do it. Consequently, the LDL particles accumulate inside the artery tissue.

Once they are trapped, the LDL particles oxidize, or decay. The white blood cells of the immune system recognize the decaying LDL as a threat to health and immediately storm down on them. The LDL particles don't belong inside your artery walls, and one way or another the immune system's cells—mostly T cells and B cells—mean to get them out of there. Under most other circumstances, the arrival of immune cells spells almost certain victory—and a restoration of health. But what the good guys don't realize is that, in this case, it's a trap.

The immune cells that enter the artery walls are called monocytes, a fairly immature type of immune-system cell. Once inside the artery, monocytes transform into much more sophisticated and powerful cells called macrophages. Macrophages are capable of destroying bacteria, viruses, and even cancer cells. They can also call out even more powerful immune cells and immune proteins, if needed.

Once the macrophages are in place, they start gobbling up the decaying LDL. Soon they are engorged with these rotting lipid balls. In fact, they are so obese with oxidized LDL that they look foamy—hence their other name, foam cells. At that point, the immune cells are rendered useless. They're essentially sick from LDL poisoning.

None of this is good, and the immune system knows it. As their last act, the macrophages call for help. Now entering the fray is a protein known as complement, a type of immune weapon that's already present in the bloodstream. Complement destroys disease-causing bacteria that are present in the blood by poking holes in them. Unfortunately, complement is not a very discriminating weapon. It can poke holes in the bacteria, yes, but it also tends to poke holes in healthy tissues, including blood vessels, triggering an even greater inflammatory reaction in the artery tissue. Blood leaks out from the artery and clots in tissues, where it will eventually be eliminated by lymph and immune cells.

Whenever there is a wound in the body, bacteria are likely to show up.

Most of us already have strains of disease-causing bacteria living in our tissues, including the types that cause pneumonia, ulcers, or even gum disease commonly known as gingivitis. These and other types of bacteria are always looking for out-of-the-way, nutrient-rich environments where they can make themselves at home. The wounds in the artery wall fit the bill nicely. Once the bacteria take up residence in the artery, an even more intense immune reaction occurs as more immune cells enter the mix, which makes the artery even more inflamed. Unfortunately, this intense inflammatory reaction only serves to make the plaque bigger, as a swarm of immune cells gobble up LDL and form a mass that protrudes through the inner lining of the artery. That swollen protrusion, called a fatty streak, is the second stage in the formation of a cholesterol plaque. As LDL continues to enter the artery wall, the fatty streak grows into a boil, or full-blown plaque.

If the amount of LDL in the artery wall were reduced, the creation of plaques would stop and the process would gradually reverse itself, because the immune system would be able to clean up the existing inflammatory mess in the artery. But because the LDL is so abundant, and because even more keeps showing up, the immune system is overwhelmed.

Inside the plaques are multitudes of white blood cells that are filled with LDL cholesterol. When these cells die, they release their cholesterol load. In time, a pool of cholesterol collects inside the plaque. Like a boil that is filled with pus, these cholesterol-filled plaques are highly unstable and prone to rupture. When a plaque does burst, the force of the rupture and the debris released by the plaque forms a wound on the artery lining.

Cardiologists refer to the inner lining of the artery as the intima. In health, the intima is a smooth, pristine surface that allows blood to flow within the artery with the least amount of resistance. But as the plaque grows, the intima becomes a bulbous, irregular surface, marked by boils and unhealed wounds. Periodically a plaque bursts open, and that's when things can get really dangerous.

First a Wound, Then a Clot— and Then a Heart Attack

Whenever a plaque bursts and spews forth its contents, it creates a wound in the intima. A wound in the artery wall is treated like any other wound in the body. Blood proteins and clotting factors arrive on the scene and, in an effort to close the wound in the artery wall, form a clot, or thrombus, over the wound. On top of the clot, a fibrous cap forms. The creation of a plaque and the opening of a wound in the artery are highly inflammatory events. Immune cells arrive, gobble up oxidized LDL and homocysteine, and start the inflammation process. This, of course, makes the artery even more inflamed. The immune cells also eat away at the fibrous cap on top of the plaque, causing it to wear away and increasing the likelihood of rupture. Repeated rupturing makes that clot get bigger, of course.

The thing that causes heart attacks is not the size of the original plaque, but the size of the blood clot that forms when the plaque erupts. A clot can become so big that it blocks blood from flowing within the artery. Or the clot can break free from the plaque and float downstream, where it can become lodged in a bottleneck in the artery, where it can block blood flow to the heart or brain and cause a heart attack or stroke. (A clot that becomes detached is called an embolus.)

Scientists used to believe that the cholesterol plaque grew to the point that it obstructed the artery entirely and thereby blocked blood flow to the heart, thus causing a heart attack. But this is not what really happens in most cases. In fact, only about 15 percent of heart attacks are caused when plaques grow to be so large that they actually obstruct the passageway in the artery.

Even small plaques can erupt and give rise to clots that are large enough to cause heart attacks. In fact, 70 percent of all heart attacks are caused by arteries that are only 30 percent closed by cholesterol plaque. An angiogram may show that only 20 to 30 percent of the artery is blocked, so 70 to 80 percent of the artery is open. Yet even such a small plaque can rupture and result in a clot large enough to close off the artery and cause a heart attack. All of this means that the size of the plaque is less important than its stability. Inflammation makes the plaque more unstable, and thus more likely to rupture. This explains why heart attacks can be sudden and often entirely unexpected.

Clots are the critical factor. You don't want them to form at all, but if they do, you don't want them to become too big. Unfortunately, the typical Western diet adversely affects the blood proteins and clotting factors in your blood and makes it much more likely that they will form large clots.

The first domino in the chain of events that leads to a heart attack is clearly LDL cholesterol. It's possible, however, that HDL protects you from heart disease because it may have an anti-inflammatory effect on arteries.

Certain drugs, among them the nonsteroidal anti-inflammatory drugs (NSAIDs) aspirin and ibuprofin, also have anti-inflammatory effects. These drugs have long been prescribed to reduce the risk of heart attack and stroke. New research suggests that these NSAIDs prevent the inflammatory process by blocking certain immune-system activities, including cyclooxygenase-2 (COX-2). It's also possible that lipid-lowering drugs called statin drugs—which are the most commonly used drugs to treat heart disease—also have an anti-inflammatory effect, which may turn out to be the primary reason for their efficacy. Studies have shown that the statin drugs have little if any effect on the size of the artery plaques—they are prescribed to lower LDL in the bloodstream—but recent research has shown that they do indeed reduce inflammation in the artery. Scientists aren't sure yet why or how they do this.

Why Heart Disease Is Often Not Diagnosed

Andrew was a 55-year-old man who was 50 pounds overweight and suffered regular chest pain, especially under even the mildest form of exertion, such as climbing a flight of stairs. His doctor ordered an angiogram, a test in which a radioactive "dye" is injected into the coronary arteries, after which X-ray images can be used to see the condition of the arteries. Angiograms reveal whether or not plaques are rising from the intima and blocking the flow of blood.

Andrew's angiogram did not find any blockages in his three main coronary arteries. Consequently, his doctor dismissed the possibility of coronary heart disease and instead treated Andrew for a possible digestive disorder. But the chest pain continued. Eventually, Andrew came to me.

After giving him a physical examination and running a battery of blood tests on him, I performed a SPECT test, the most advanced form of diagnostic technology available to cardiologists. SPECT cameras provide extremely precise information on how much blood is flowing to the heart under varying degrees of stress, or the absence of stress. The camera revealed that Andrew did indeed have coronary heart disease, but it was not the type that would turn up on an angiogram. Angiograms can only reveal plaques that grow on the intima and project out into the passageway of the artery, known as the lumen (the cavity of a tubular organ). They cannot see disease that is growing within the artery tissue.

Thus, though Andrew's coronary problem could not be revealed by angiogram, that did not mean that he was well. On the contrary, he did have significant heart disease and in fact was a likely candidate for a heart attack. Andrew didn't have lumen disease, as the angiogram correctly showed. He had artery disease, which the angiogram couldn't see. Both lumen disease and artery disease have the same cause, but only one can be seen by an angiogram.

I took Andrew off all the medication for a digestive disorder, placed him on a drug for chest pain, and instructed him on how to follow Phase 1 of the Fleming Program. I followed him closely for the next year. Three months later, he no longer had chest pain. Nine months later, he had lost 50 pounds and was off all medication.

How Cholesterol Becomes Elevated

Coronary heart disease, both lumen and artery disease, begins when LDL cholesterol becomes excessive in the bloodstream. There are a number of causes of this. LDL levels rise when we eat too much saturated fat, the type that's found primarily in animal foods such as red meat, dairy products, eggs, and chicken. Another way to raise your blood cholesterol is simply to eat too many calories, whether the source is fats, sugars, or carbohydrates. Excess calories raise triglycerides, a percentage of which become LDL cholesterol. Coffee also appears to elevate your blood cholesterol, and in some people it can raise it significantly, by 10 percent or more. Two substances in coffee appear to be the culprits, caffestol and kahweol. For a time it was thought that these substances were fully eliminated in filtered coffee, but a study done by Danish researchers and published in the *American Journal of Clinical Nutrition* (Christensen 2001) found that four cups or more of filtered coffee per day increased both cholesterol and homocysteine levels. Unfiltered coffee had been shown to raise cholesterol consistently, but this recent study demonstrated that even four cups of filtered coffee raises cholesterol and homocysteine.

Fats

Fat can increase your cholesterol directly, by means of saturated fat, or indirectly, by means of elevated calories. Therefore, we should take a closer look at fat and its sources. Fat is the most calorically dense substance in the food supply. A gram of fat contains 9 calories, whereas a gram of carbohydrate and a gram of protein each contains 4 calories. There are four types of fat, and each affects your blood cholesterol differently.

SATURATED FATS

Saturated fat is called "saturated," because it is filled to capacity, saturated, with hydrogen atoms. It is solid at room temperature, and is found mostly in animal foods, with the exception of fish, which is typically low in saturated fat. It raises LDL cholesterol levels and substantially increases your risk of cancer, overweight, obesity, and other serious illnesses.

In Phase 1 of my diet, all saturated fat is eliminated in order to bring down LDL cholesterol levels rapidly. In Phase 2, up to 5 grams of saturated fat are allowed per day.

As you will see from the table on pages 31–33, the major sources of fat, and specifically saturated fat, are beef, pork, lamb, and chicken. Most fish has negligible amounts of fat, the primary exception being salmon, which is rich in a type of polyunsaturated fat that boosts the immune system. Whole milk and cheese can also be major sources of fat. Milk and milk products (discussed in chapter 6) should be avoided in Phase 1 and eaten only in small amounts, if at all, in Phase 2. (I make this recommendation because milk can be highly inflammatory, which means it promotes heart disease and other illnesses in ways that go beyond the issue of fat.)

HYDROGENATED FATS

Hydrogenated fats are basically saturated fats that are created when vegetable fats, which are ordinarily liquid, are stuffed with hydrogen atoms so that they will be solids at room temperature. These fats, often called trans-fatty acids or trans-fats, appear most commonly as margarine and in processed foods, fast foods, and baked products. Because these fats are saturated, they raise LDL cholesterol.

I recommend that you avoid hydrogenated fats entirely.

POLYUNSATURATED FATS

Polyunsaturated fats are not as saturated or filled with hydrogen atoms as saturated fats. This makes polyunsaturated fats liquid at room temperature.

Number of Calories, and Fat Content (in grams) of Animal Foods

MEAT ✳ 99.2 g (3.5 oz.), Roasted or Broiled

	Calories	Total Fat (grams)	Saturated Fat (grams)
Beef			
Regular ground beef	289	21	8
Lean ground beef (93% lean)	272	18	7
Bottom round prime	249	13	5
Ribs, whole	280	19	8
Short ribs, choice	295	18	8
Sirloin, prime	237	12	5
Pork			
Bacon	576	49	17
Boston butt, fresh (from the shoulder)	273	16	6
Canadian bacon	185	8	3
Center rib, boneless	214	10	4
Ground pork	297	21	8
Ham, canned, extra lean	136	5	2
Ham, cured, lean	157	6	2
Loin, whole	187	8	3
Tenderloin	164	5	2
Lamb, trimmed			
Lamb, leg	191	8	3
Chicken			
Breast with skin	197	8	4
Breast, without skin	165	4	1
Dark meat, with skin	253	16	4
Dark meat, without skin	205	10	3
Leg, with skin	216	11	3
Leg, without skin	172	6	1
Light meat, with skin	222	11	3
Light meat, without skin	173	6	1
Turkey			
Breast, with skin	153	3	1

(continued)

Turkey (continued)

	Calories	Total Fat (grams)	Saturated Fat (grams)
Breast, without skin	135	1	<1
Dark meat, with skin	182	7	2
Dark meat, without skin	162	4	1
Leg, with skin	170	5	2
Leg, without skin	159	4	1
Light meat, with skin	164	5	1
Light meat, without skin	140	1	<1
Wing, with skin	207	10	3
Wing, without skin	163	3	1

DAIRY ✳ ½ cup (113 ml. or 4 oz.)

Milk and Milk Products

Whole milk	64	4	2
Low-fat (2%)	50	2	1
Low-fat (1%)	42	1	1
Skim milk	35	<1	<1
Buttermilk, low-fat	40	1	<1
Heavy cream	354	37	23
Sour cream	214	21	13
Half and half	130	12	7

Cheese

Blue cheese	353	29	19
Brie	334	28	17
Camembert	300	24	15
Cheddar	403	33	21
Cottage cheese, low-fat	72	1	<1
Cream cheese	349	35	22
Feta	264	21	15
Monterey Jack	373	30	19
Mozzarella, part-skim	280	17	11
Parmesan	392	26	16
Ricotta, part-skim	138	8	5

(continued)

Cheese (continued)			
	Calories	**Total Fat** (grams)	**Saturated Fat** (grams)
Roquefort	369	31	19
Swiss	376	28	18
Yogurt			
Plain, low fat	63	2	1
Fruit, low-fat	99	1	1
Whole-milk	61	3	2

FISH ✳ 99.2 g (3½ oz.), Roasted or Broiled

Bass, freshwater	153	5	1
Bluefish	166	6	1
Carp	162	7	1
Cod	105	1	<1
Flounder	117	2	<1
Haddock	112	1	<1
Halibut	140	3	<1
Herring	203	12	3
Mackerel	262	18	4
Orange roughy	169	9	<1
Red snapper	128	2	<1
Salmon	216	11	2
Sea bass	124	3	1
Shad	263	18	6
Shark	174	6	1
Swordfish	155	5	1
Trout, rainbow	151	4	1
Tuna, bluefin	184	6	2
Tuna, yellowfin	145	1	<1

Technically, a fat is referred to as "polyunsaturated" when it lacks four or more hydrogen atoms in its molecular makeup. Monounsaturated fats have slightly more hydrogen atoms than polys, but they, too, are unsaturated and therefore liquid at room temperature. Polyunsaturated fats are oils that are pressed from whole grains, nuts, seeds, vegetables, and fish. Some of these polyunsaturated fats can lower blood cholesterol levels somewhat, but the effect on your body depends on the type that you eat.

Polyunsaturated fats are commonly divided into omega-3 and omega-6 fatty acids, terms that refer to features of the molecules that make up these oils. Omega-3 fatty acids, found in fish, flaxseeds, flax oil, almonds, and walnuts, boost the immune system and reduce inflammation and thus reduce your risk of inflammatory illnesses.

Omega-6 fatty acids come from trans-fatty acids and many vegetable oils, such as corn oil. Studies have shown that omega-6 fatty acids, along with the oils that they come in, rapidly oxidize, or decay, which means they produce more oxidants, or free radicals, than other oils. They become rancid. This rapid oxidation also transforms LDL and homocysteine into highly toxic substances in your arteries, which in turn promotes inflammation throughout the body, including the arteries that lead to the heart and brain. Moreover, every food or substance that promotes oxidation causes cells and tissues to break down and age. Organs shrink and the DNA in cells can become deformed, thus increasing the chances of cancer.

Many physicians and laypeople have come to believe that, since the omega-3s lower blood cholesterol and boost the immune system, they should be used as supplements. I strongly disagree with this, however. First, all fats are calorically dense, meaning that they add calories to your diet. The more calories you eat, the more likely you are to gain weight. Excess weight is highly inflammatory. So, too, are diets rich in calories. Excess calorie consumption is pro-inflammatory, which substantially raises the likelihood that it will promote serious illnesses. Do not eat excess calories, no matter where they come from. This is especially important when it comes to consuming any form of fat, including omega-3 fatty acids. As long as you get them in food, you won't have any problem, but supplements of fat can be dangerous.

MONOUNSATURATED FATS

Monounsaturated fats, found in olives, nuts, and seeds, are much more "stable" than polyunsaturated fats, which means that they do not oxidize as rapidly. Olive oil, which contains oleic acid, tends to resist oxidation even when you heat it. There is also some evidence that monounsaturated fats protect against cancer, and olive oil is rich in phytochemicals that boost immune function.

Monounsaturated fats do not raise or lower your total cholesterol level, but they may increase your HDL somewhat. During Phase 2 of my program, up to 15 percent of the diet may be derived from fat. I recommend that you limit saturated fat to 5 grams per day, and that you limit polyunsaturated and monounsaturated fat to 10 grams per day for a total of 15 grams of fat per day. However, I do encourage people to have vegetarian days in which they eat no saturated fat, in which case they can increase their intake of poly- and monounsaturated fats to a total of 15 grams. In chapter 14, I provide numerous recipes for their healthy use.

Triglycerides: Cholesterol's Accomplice

Triglycerides, three fatty-acid chains attached to a glycerol molecule, have long been thought of as a secondary factor in the cause of heart disease. For decades, physicians routinely dismissed triglyceride levels in the blood as having little importance, and, to be fair, the research was equivocal on their role in the etiology of heart disease.

Today we know that triglycerides are important because about 20 percent of your blood's total triglyceride content becomes LDL cholesterol. That means that the higher your triglycerides, the higher your LDL cholesterol is going to be, and the greater your risk of heart attack or stroke.

We also know that triglycerides play a major role in metabolic syndrome, the constellation of factors that includes overweight, high insulin, high glucose, high LDL cholesterol, and high triglycerides. All of these factors lead to type 2 diabetes (often referred to as adult-onset diabetes), claudication (insufficient blood circulation in the legs), and heart attacks. (Metabolic syndrome, diabetes, and the role played by triglycerides are discussed in greater detail in the next chapter.)

Triglyceride levels are raised by saturated fat and excess calories, including those that come from processed foods, sugar, and excess intake of fruit. All of these foods contain lots of calories, and thereby increase triglycerides and LDL. They also do it quickly. If a doctor draws blood from you within an hour of your consumption of a high-fat, high-calorie meal, your blood will look cloudy—in some cases, even white—from the amount of fats in your blood. Many of these blood fats adhere to your red blood cells, causing them to become sticky. Red blood cells are similar in shape to Lifesaver candy: They are round and have a small indentation in the center where they carry oxygen, and when they become sticky, they adhere to one another, resembling a roll of coins. This condition, called the "rouleaux effect," prevents the red cells from taking up as much oxygen as they otherwise could. It also prevents them from circulating freely throughout the capillary system. Red blood cells are about 7.5 microns in diameter. Many tiny capillaries are as small as 3.5 microns in diameter. In health, the red blood cells bend and fold in order to pass freely through these tiny vessels, so they can bring oxygen to cells that are lined up along the edge of the capillary. But when the red blood cells become sticky from excess triglycerides and adhere to one another, they face a dilemma, much like a bus that attempts to drive on a bicycle path: there's simply no room to squeeze through! As a result, all the cells that are waiting for the arrival of their oxygen supply begin to suffocate. Eventually, as these cells die, tissue withers and shrinks. The remaining healthy, functional portions of organs get smaller, and aging is accelerated. Cells need oxygen to survive, so we need to maintain healthy circulation. High triglycerides reduce circulation throughout the body.

For all of these reasons, it's essential to keep triglycerides down. A safe triglyceride level is 150 mg/dL or lower.

Stress and Cholesterol Levels

Stress is another cause of elevated blood cholesterol levels, including LDL cholesterol. Several different factors related to stress drive this phenomenon. The heart's preferred fuel is fat. Evolution has trained us to react to stress either by fighting or fleeing the perceived threat in the environment. In order to fight or flee, the heart has to work harder, which means it's going to need more fuel. Once the body is thrown into stress, certain hormones, particularly cortisol, force the release of fat stored in the tissues, which floods the bloodstream and flows to the heart. That, of course, increases blood cholesterol levels, including LDL cholesterol. The problem is that stress tends to be chronic in our society. We don't fight or flee when confronted by many of the experiences we regard as threatening. Also, many people who suffer from chronic stress do not exercise, but instead live sedentary lifestyles. That means that the heart doesn't utilize the available fat as fuel in order to fight, flee, or simply burn as a fuel for exercise. On the contrary, once the fat is dumped into the bloodstream, its primary effect is to contribute to coronary heart disease, which ends up destroying the heart.

Stress is yet another reason why exercise is so important. You're going to be under stress from time to time, so your heart had better utilize that fat as fuel, rather than being poisoned by it.

An Ideal Blood Cholesterol Level

The most important number in your cholesterol profile is the number for your total cholesterol, including both LDL and HDL. An ideal total cholesterol level is 150 mg/dL or lower. We know that that's the benchmark for health because the research shows that people who have cholesterol levels of 150 or lower experience extremely low rates of heart disease, heart attacks, and strokes.

Do not be content if your doctor says your cholesterol level is "normal" or in the "healthy range." Normal is not healthy. It's important for you to know the actual numbers. Many physicians consider 190 or 200 mg/dL a normal cholesterol level and will tell their patients that their cholesterol is fine. In fact, numbers like these are not fine and can put you very much at risk for a heart attack or stroke. According to the Framingham Heart Study and other research, the rate of heart attacks starts to go up sharply when cholesterol levels rise above 180 mg/dL. On the other hand, cholesterol levels of 150 or less have been consistently shown to be safe.

Average cholesterol levels among Americans are above 210 mg/dL, which I consider an extremely dangerous risk and in need of immediate treatment. Heart disease is now the number one killer in the United States, and in the entire Western world. Every day, many people with cholesterol levels below 210 have heart attacks.

Cholesterol level is but one indicator and should be considered within a constellation of tests (more about this in chapter 9). Besides the cholesterol test, the most important test is a C-RP (C-reactive protein) test because it measures the extent of the inflammation in your body. You should also get your triglyceride level tested. If your cholesterol and triglyceride levels are 150 or lower and your C-RP is low, you are very likely in good shape. The results of other tests, such as homocysteine and those I mention in chapter 8, should also be examined carefully.

After considering your total cholesterol level, you'll want to examine your LDL and HDL profiles. An ideal LDL cholesterol is under 100 mg/dL and preferably less than 70, and HDL should be 50 or above. HDL is increased in your bloodstream by exercise, by behaviors that reduce stress, and by certain foods, including small amounts of alcoholic beverages such as beer and wine. People with low *total* cholesterol numbers can have low HDL and still be in excellent health, however.

Low HDL is often present among people who eat a low-fat diet and have low total cholesterol. For example, among the Tarahumara Indians of northern Mexico, most have total cholesterol levels that are below 150. They also have low HDLs, many as low as 15. Yet the Tarahumara have virtually no heart disease, diabetes, or high blood pressure. They eat a diet that's essentially a high-carbohydrate, low-fat regimen. As long as they remain on that diet, they remain healthy. They also get plenty of exercise. The men play a game similar to soccer, only it requires more than 100 miles of running. The women play the game, too, but they run only 60 miles. Despite all that running, they still have low HDL levels. But the truth is, the Tarahumaras' total cholesterol levels are so low that they don't need much HDL to protect their hearts.

People with high cholesterol levels often console themselves with the fact that they have plenty of "good cholesterol." They shouldn't be so sanguine. HDL levels tend to be higher among those who have high total cholesterols, and these people are still very much at risk for a heart attack. I believe that when total cholesterol rises to dangerous levels, the body may increase production of HDL as way of protecting itself against sudden death. But high HDL cannot stave off the effects of total cholesterol of 200 or higher.

HDL Ratio: More Form Than Substance

No doubt you have heard cardiologists refer to the cholesterol-to-HDL ratio, or HDL ratio for short, as an important diagnostic tool for determining your risk of heart attacks. If your total cholesterol is 200 and your HDL is 50, the total cholesterol is four times the HDL and you have a ratio of 4 to 1, usually written 4:1. If your cholesterol level is 300 and your HDL is 50, you would have a ratio of 6:1. If your total cholesterol level is 150 and your HDL is 50, your ratio would be 3:1.

Cardiologists maintain that anyone with a ratio of 4:1 or higher is at high risk of having a heart attack. I do not support the whole ratio concept, for the simple reason that people could have a high ratio even if they had low cholesterol and low HDLs—and they often do. Many of the Tarahumaras, for example, have total cholesterol levels of 150 mg/dL and HDLs of 15 mg/dL, giving them a ratio of 10:1, which would seem to represent extremely high risk of heart attack. Fortunately, for the Tarahumara, that's not the case, and the ratio is meaningless. Conversely, people with total cholesterol levels of 250 and HDLs of 75 have a ratio below 4:1, which should indicate good health and low risk, but a total cholesterol of 250 represents anything but good health.

When it comes to cholesterol levels, you should place the most emphasis on your total cholesterol number. That will give you the clearest picture of your risk.

Nevertheless, as I stress throughout this book, cholesterol is only one piece in an extremely complex picture. A cholesterol level of 180 or higher is high enough to combine with the other 11 risk factors to create a dangerous inflammatory reaction inside your arteries. Once that process is under way, it can create highly volatile plaques that can erupt and form life-threatening clots. You only need so much cholesterol to create those plaques, especially if other risk factors, such as homocysteine or fibrinogen, are elevated.

How to Lower Blood Cholesterol and Reverse Heart Disease

The first step in reversing heart disease is to substantially reduce your cholesterol and trigylceride levels, preferably to 150 mg/dL or lower. If your cholesterol level is 210 or higher, a significant drop in cholesterol may cause reversal, even if you don't get it down to 150. But at 150, reversal is a virtual guarantee.

There are five dependable ways of lowering blood cholesterol and triglycerides.

1. If you smoke, stop. Cigarette, cigar, and pipe smoking elevate LDL cholesterol levels dramatically and create atherosclerotic plaque. Cigarette smoking is among the most important causes of heart disease, cancer, and diseases of the lungs.

2. Reduce or eliminate saturated fat from your diet. The Phase 1 diet eliminates all saturated fat, which is one reason why it causes such precipitous drops in blood cholesterol. Phase 2 allows 5 grams of fat per day, which is low enough to reduce cholesterol levels and protect your heart.

3. Lower your caloric intake, especially from fat and processed foods. Phases 1 and 2 eliminate processed carbohydrates from the diet, as well as most forms of fat. This causes calories to drop dramatically and results in significant and healthful weight loss. The weight reduction causes rapid declines in blood cholesterol and triglycerides, which affect your LDL levels for the better.

4. Eat a high-fiber diet. Soluble fibers found in whole grains such as brown rice, oats, and barley lower blood cholesterol. Phase 2 of the Fleming Program includes lots of whole grains.

5. Eat antioxidant-rich foods and take an antioxidant supplement, especially during Phase 1 of the program. Studies have shown that vitamin C lowers cholesterol and causes few if any side effects. I recommend up to 500 mg of vitamin C a day, along with a vitamin C–rich diet. Phase 1 is an antioxidant-rich diet that's especially abundant in vitamin C.

Researchers have found that 200 IU per day of vitamin E taken for four weeks can lower total cholesterol by 15 percent and LDL cholesterol by 8 percent.

I have also included an option of using herbs to lower cholesterol. The Fleming Program uses all of these methods optimally. I do not stress cholesterol-lowering herbs; however, certain plants—specifically garlic, gugulipid, and hawthorn—do appear to lower cholesterol, and I sometimes suggest that they be used as an adjunct to the program, or as flavor enhancers in your cooking. These herbs appear to act on the liver to reduce LDL and increase HDL production.

Some studies suggest that garlic can lower cholesterol levels and protect cholesterol from being oxidized, and oxidation is what triggers the inflammatory process. Garlic may inhibit clot formation as well. I don't rely on any herb to lower cholesterol substantially, but do use garlic as a flavor enhancer in my food whenever it seems appropriate. For those who want to use garlic as a supplement, you can eat a clove a day or take garlic powder, such as kyolic.

Studies have shown that gugulipid, an extract of the Indian tree *Commiphora mukul*, can lower cholesterol by 21 percent and triglycerides by 25 percent in just three to eight weeks. The extract also raises HDL by 60 percent in patients studied. Gugulipid is available in natural-foods and health-food stores. The standard dosage is 500 mg, taken three times per day. No adverse effects have been shown to date.

Hawthorn (*Crataegus oxyacantha*), a spiny plant that grows throughout Europe, has been shown to reduce angina pain in humans and lower cholesterol and reverse atherosclerosis in animal studies. Standard doses range from 100 to 200 mg per day. No adverse side effects have been found.

The Phase 1 and 2 diets are the real source of health. In fact, no other program has proved to be as effective as the Fleming diet for reversing heart disease. The Fleming Program has been scientifically documented to show reversal of heart disease in 100 percent of the people who have followed it. Other regimens claim to reverse heart disease, but only this program has been shown to do it without medication and in all study participants who adhered to the program.

Here's how the program causes the reversal of cholesterol-plaque formation. When you lower blood cholesterol, you force the body to utilize the cholesterol that it has in reserve, from all sources, including the pools of cholesterol in the plaques themselves.

The body uses cholesterol to create hormones such as estrogen and testosterone, cell membranes, and bile acids and to metabolize vitamin D. Your body needs a certain amount of cholesterol to carry out these functions, so if you stop eating saturated fat and excess calories, the amount of cholesterol it has to work with drops precipitously. That forces the body to call on its reserves in its muscles and arteries in order to maintain normal function. Don't worry. You've got more than enough cholesterol stored in your tissues to meet your body's needs for many years to come. In fact, only about 7 percent of the total cholesterol load is in your blood. The other 93 percent is stored in your tissues. In addition, your liver produces about 1,000 mg of cholesterol a day. Most of that is utilized by the body or eliminated in the feces.

When your body is deprived of excess cholesterol, it is forced to draw the cholesterol out of the plaques. This does two important things: First, it causes the plaques to shrink, opening your arteries and allowing blood to flow more freely. Second, without the pool of cholesterol inside, the plaques stabilize, so they are less likely to rupture. In essence, you have taken yourself out of jeopardy of having a heart attack.

You might think that it takes a long time for these two steps to occur, but on my program, both of these goals can be met within the first week or two. That means that after a few days of living on Phase 1, you are forcing your body to utilize its cholesterol reserves, and thus forcing it to use up the cholesterol in the plaques. As the plaques shrink, the inflammatory reaction cools and the arteries start to heal. You are now reversing your coronary heart disease.

Why Drugs Don't Cure Heart Disease

The essential point to understand is that in order to reverse heart disease, you have to reduce the overall quantity of cholesterol in your body. When you've done that, you will create a cholesterol-deprived environment, and your body will be forced to utilize the cholesterol in your plaques. That's going to make them shrink.

I emphasize this point because it also reveals why cholesterol-lowering drugs fail to cure heart disease, even though they lower blood cholesterol. The way the most commonly used cholesterol-lowering medications work is by causing the liver to produce less cholesterol. Many cells produce some cholesterol, but the liver by far produces the most. By lowering the cholesterol output of the liver, these drugs reduce the amount of cholesterol in the blood, but not enough to force your body to draw on its reserves. There's still plenty of cholesterol in your tissues, which is where the body needs it to metabolize vitamin D, create bile acids, and produce cell membranes. All that's happened is that there's less in your bloodstream. Meanwhile, the drop in blood cholesterol is not all that much—certainly not enough to create a cholesterol-deprived environment in your body, and therefore not enough to force your body to draw on the cholesterol in the plaques. Meanwhile, you're probably still putting enough saturated fat in your mouth to maintain the overall cholesterol level in your body, meaning that the change in blood cholesterol is largely a cosmetic improvement, not a particularly therapeutic one.

Many scientists—and I am one of them—now believe that the reason the cholesterol-lowering medications—namely, the statin drugs—are able to protect your blood vessels and reduce your risk of having a heart attack is that they have an anti-inflammatory effect. As I said earlier, drug treatment alone is not sufficient to reverse the disease. All it will do, at best, is postpone it.

A Revolutionary Idea: Cure the Illness, Don't Just Manage It

By adopting the Fleming Program, you will reduce your cholesterol level substantially. One of the goals of Phase 1 is to reduce your cholesterol to 150 mg/dL or lower, and it can be accomplished in a relatively short time. Another goal of the overall program is to get you off medication. When you think about it, that's a revolutionary approach to health care. Most people on cholesterol-lowering medication or any cardiovascular drug are expected to remain on their pills for the rest of their lives. I do not have such a pessimistic approach to the treatment of heart disease. I expect my program not only to protect my patients from a heart attack or a stroke but actually to strengthen their hearts and their overall health. Yes, I often prescribe medication at the outset of the treatment. But inevitably I take people off their drugs. Why? Because their health improves so dramatically that they no longer need them.

The Truth About Gaining Weight

WHEN HE CAME TO SEE ME IN OCTOBER 2000, Jim, a six-foot, 48-year-old computer expert, weighed 306 pounds, and all his numbers were off the charts. His total cholesterol level was 240 mg/dL, his triglyceride level was 453 mg/dL. His homocysteine was 13.4 µmol/L (4 to 12 is normal in men, and 4 to 10 is normal in women); fibrinogen, 495 (the normal range is 200 to 400); and his lipoprotein (a), a protein produced by the liver that promotes the creation of clots, was 58 (normal is less than 30). All of this suggested rampant inflammation throughout his body, but especially in his arteries, and at 3.01 mg/dL, Jim's C-reactive protein level reflected that. On top of all of this, Jim was diabetic and on oral medication. In short, he was a heart attack waiting to happen.

While I was examining him, Jim told me that he didn't eat much fat. "Really, I don't believe I eat much fat, Doc," he said. "I try to avoid too much meat because it constipates me. And whenever I eat a muffin or something like that, I always make sure it's fat-free. I also try to eat whole-wheat muffins and whole-wheat bread. I thought whole grains were good for me. What's going on?"

"Jim, the first thing to understand is that whole-wheat bread and whole-wheat muffins are not whole grains," I said. "They're processed foods—the same as white bread or white rolls. And all processed foods cause people to gain weight.

"For a grain to be considered whole, it must be unaltered from its original state," I continued. "It's got to be in the same state that nature made it. Whole grains are amaranth, brown rice, barley, millet, corn, quinoa, wheat berries—there are lots of them. They have not been milled, or cracked, or altered by some form of processing. That means they're still nutritionally intact."

"Okay, but what's wrong with whole-wheat bread, or any processed food?" Jim asked. "Especially processed foods that don't contain fat? I mean, I thought fat was the bad thing. Isn't that what they've been telling us for years now?"

"Yes, you're right, Jim," I said. "What they failed to tell you is that processed foods are just as bad as fat when it comes to weight gain, maybe worse. Processed foods are packed with excess calories. Ounce for ounce, there are more calories in bread than there are in a steak, as long as the fat's been trimmed from the steak. Did you know that? There are about three times as many calories, ounce for ounce, in Oreo cookies as in pork tenderloin."

"I can't believe it!" Jim said.

"It's true. Processed foods give your body more calories than it can burn. And the calories that you don't burn, you store as fat. There are other reasons why processed foods are bad for you," I continued. "The carbohydrates in processed foods are rapidly absorbed by the body, which means they drive up your insulin levels. High insulin leads to heart disease, diabetes, and many other disorders."

"I try to avoid fat, and now I have to stay away from bread and other processed foods," Jim said. "What do I have to do? Starve?"

"No, Jim," I said. "You can eat to your heart's content, as long as you eat foods that are unprocessed, low in calories, and rich in nutrition and fiber. These foods will reduce your weight, lower your insulin levels, and create a new healthy version of yourself."

Like many people who are ready to change their lives and regain their health, Jim adhered to Phase 1 of the Fleming Program to the letter. And as we both had hoped, the program changed his life. In less than a year, Jim's weight dropped to 191, a loss of more than 100 pounds. His cholesterol fell to 169 mg/dL, his triglycerides to 160 mg/dL, and his C-RP was 0.4 mg/dL. Jim's homocysteine went down to 9 µmol/L, and his lipoprotein (a) dropped to 30. His blood sugar stabilized, he was no longer diabetic, and I was able to take him off his diabetes medication. I followed Jim closely for a year: His weight remained at 190 and his numbers all stayed well within the healthy ranges. He was in excellent health. But that doesn't begin to explain all that it did for his life, health, self-image, and longevity. He told me on numerous occasions, "This program saved my life."

Why It's So Easy to Gain Weight on a Typical Modern Diet

According to the Centers for Disease Control (CDC), more than 60 percent of American adults and 13 percent of American children are overweight. The consequences of this epidemic are catastrophic. The list of illnesses that being overweight triggers is both long and terrifying: heart disease, many forms of cancer, diabetes, arthritis, blindness, gangrene, kidney disease, gout, high blood pressure, gallstones, sleep disturbances, reproductive problems, and incontinence, to name just a handful. The U.S. surgeon general has reported that the health-care costs associated with overweight and obesity are now greater than those for cigarette smokers. Dutch researchers recently reported (Wannamethee 2002) that people who are overweight at the age of 40 die three years younger, on average, than their lean counterparts.

Meanwhile, more people than ever before are becoming overweight at younger ages. And just as with adults, illnesses related to overweight—high blood pressure, diabetes (a metabolic disorder), and heart disease—among children are skyrocketing. Up until recently, type 2 diabetes (often referred to as adult-onset diabetes) was rare in children and young people. But in the last five years, the CDC has reported a tenfold increase in the number of children with diabetes. On top of this, of course, is the incalculable psychological suffering that occurs in people who are overweight, especially children.

The most common consequences of overweight are heart disease and type 2 diabetes—in fact, these three conditions tend to go hand in hand. People who are overweight often have high glucose, high insulin, high cholesterol, high triglycerides, and coronary heart disease and are either borderline or full-blown diabetics. As many as 90 percent of diabetics are overweight, and the majority of them will die of heart disease.

For these reasons, most overweight people today report being on a diet, or are trying to lose weight. In fact, many overweight adults and children will tell you that they eat as little as they can. But as the statistics bear out, they are not succeeding on their diets. Ironically, many people report being constantly hungry from dieting but at the same time are still gaining weight! How is this possible? you may ask. The answer is that they eat too many processed foods. In fact, processed foods play a major role in causing overweight, heart disease, and diabetes.

Processed foods are those that have been altered from the way nature created them or have been produced almost entirely from artificial ingredients by food manufacturers. Processed foods include sugar, syrups, bread (all forms), rolls, crackers, chips, cookies, muffins, pastries, waffles, pancakes, Jell-O, puddings, candy, soda pop, fruit juices, cereals, hot dogs, sausage, SPAM, dehydrated foods, most canned or packaged foods, and some frozen foods. Look down any aisle of your supermarket, and, with the exception of the produce aisle and the fish and meat counters, you will see nothing but processed foods. When you think about it, processed foods make up the majority of the foods most people eat today.

Essentially, processing takes an enormous amount of food and concentrates it into a much smaller volume. The result is a food that is usually loaded with calories. For example, food manufacturers take many pounds of potatoes and turn them into a single pound of chips. Or they take pounds of wheat berries and turn them into a loaf of bread. In both cases, the calories in all those potatoes or wheat berries get distilled into that small quantity of chips or flour. You couldn't eat ten pounds of potatoes—at least not in a single sitting—but you can eat a pound of chips.

One large potato provides about 200 calories, and when you eat a potato, you're full, or close to it. Even if you ate a whole pound of potatoes—and you would really be stuffed—you would only be getting 490 calories. But a standard, one-pound bag of chips, which many people eat in a single sitting, provides 2,400 calories.

A pound of cooked wheat berries (as whole-wheat grains are called) provides about 230 calories, but a pound of bread provides about 1,200 calories.

Take those wheat kernels, remove their "germ" and hull, and grind them even finer (so that you can pack even more calories into that little bit of food), and you'll have the flour to make pretzels, a pound of which provides more than 1,700 calories.

When they process foods, manufacturers start with a quantity of unprocessed, whole food—one that contains a relatively small amount of calories—and grind it into tiny particles. Then they cook it, add sugar or fat or both, and then dry it. What they come up with is a food whose calories are concentrated into a small volume. When you eat that small volume of food, you get lots of calories, which means that even a little food can add a lot of weight.

The processed carbohydrates alone are an enormous source of calories, but when you add fat to the food, which is the case with most cookies, chips, and pastries, the calories skyrocket. Oreo cookies, for example, contain hydrogenated fats and more than 2,000 calories per pound (about 30 cookies). The standard granola bar, which many people think of as "health food," is a stealth bomber, coming in at 2,300 calories per pound.

The tables on page 49 show the number of calories in one pound of whole, unprocessed foods (such as potatoes, corn, wheat berries, brown rice, and various vegetables) and in one pound of processed foods (such as cookies, chips, and cold cereals). Notice what happens when you take a pound of, say, wheat berries and turn them into a pound of shredded wheat cereal. Or if you process those wheat berries even more and turn them into a pound of fat-free crackers. If you add fat to the flour and make cookies, you'll get an even more calorically rich food, such as Oreo cookies.

The Typical Diet

On the typical American diet, you fill your stomach with calories, not nutrition. As you probably know, it doesn't take much of an appetite to eat half a bag, or even a full bag, of chips or pretzels. You sit down in front of the television set and start eating cookies and all of a sudden you realize that you've eaten the entire box. Two thousand calories! That's more than most people need for the entire day.

In addition to being loaded with calories, processed foods contribute to weight gain by loading your blood with simple sugars. The carbohydrates in

Calories in One Pound of Unprocessed Food	
Black beans	600
Yams	525
Brown rice	500
Potatoes	490
Buckwheat groats	420
Corn	390
Oatmeal	280
Apples	270
Wheat berries	230
Strawberries	140
Broccoli	130
Lettuce	65

Calories in One Pound of Processed Food	
Corn chips	2,450
Potato chips	2,400
Popcorn with flavored oil	2,270
Oreo cookies	2,200
Dietetic cookies	2,180
Chocolate-chip cookies	2,140
Cornflakes	1,770
Popcorn, plain	1,730
Fat-free whole-wheat crackers	1,620
Shredded wheat	1,610
Entenmann's fat-free cookies	1,510
Whole-wheat bread	1,280

processed foods are actually simple, free-floating sugars. Those sugars are rapidly absorbed by your small intestine, and your bloodstream is flooded with glucose, or blood sugar. Your brain recognizes that flood of sugar as excessive and starts defensive action to decrease the blood sugar. First, it turns off your appetite. Your brain doesn't want you adding any more sugar to the blood, so essentially it tells you to stop eating. Second, the brain orders the pancreas to produce an abundance of insulin, the hormone that permits blood sugar to enter cells and be utilized as fuel. If the blood is filled with insulin, your body retains all the fat in your tissues instead of releasing it to be burned as fuel. It also stores the new fat arriving in your food. Which means you're gaining weight. Here's how it works.

Each of your cells needs only so much sugar—fuel—to function. In fact, your cells resist absorbing more sugar than they actually need. When you eat a processed food, you consume more fuel than your body needs, and this creates a big problem for your body. It needs to get rid of the extra fuel, but how? The body has two choices: to burn or to store the extra fuel. It tries to do both.

The body will burn all the calories it can, as fast as it can, but its ability to burn excess calories is limited, especially if you don't exercise. So the reality is that, without exercise, the body can't burn enough of the excess calories. Instead, your body has to store them as fat. Since processed foods provide many more calories than your body needs, they are constantly being stored as fat. Hence, two thirds of the American population is overweight.

Weight Gain and Cravings

It's possible to crave food even when you're full. That sounds hard to believe, but it happens all the time. What people don't realize is that they're not craving calories, they're craving nutrition.

Your body requires vitamins and minerals to function properly. As you know, processed foods are usually deficient in nutrition and fiber. They also lack immune-boosting phytochemicals and fiber, which your body also needs to maintain health. When you eat a quantity of, say, chips or cookies, you're getting lots of calories, but only a small quantity of nutrients. Your body still needs the nutrients to function. That means that you'll be craving food that gives you nutrition, even though you just filled up on foods that are loaded with calories. You're gaining weight but you're still hungry. Unfortunately, everything else you eat to get that nutrition will only add more calories.

Processed food, as we have seen, creates sudden steep rises and falls in blood sugar. When blood sugar is high, appetite is often turned off. Still, excess blood sugar is regarded by the brain as an emergency situation and a threat to the body's survival. In an effort to get rid of that excess blood sugar, the body burns as much fuel as possible, as rapidly as it can. Consequently, blood sugar drops off quickly. When blood sugar reaches a low ebb, hunger is turned on again. Why? Because you need more fuel to function and survive. At that point, you start craving foods that will rapidly increase your blood sugar. And you know what those are: more processed foods. So highly processed foods packed with sugar result in sudden rises and falls in blood-sugar levels and increased cravings for more processed foods.

The net effect is to be constantly craving foods that ultimately cause weight gain and sickness. This is precisely what's happening to so many children every day of their lives. They crave the foods that make them fat. Meanwhile, those same foods are not giving them adequate nutrition and fiber, which means they are also craving nutrition but don't know it. Hence, they satisfy their cravings for sugar and nutrition with low-nutrient, processed foods. The effect of that cycle is overweight, obesity, and illness, including heart disease.

It's important to remember that processed foods are only part of the formula for weight gain. The other part is dietary fat. Fat is the most calorically dense substance in the food supply, far outweighing carbohydrates and protein in its calorie density (9 calories per gram of fat, versus 4 with carbs and protein). Many processed foods are laced with fat, which make them especially weight producing. But animal foods such as cheese, whole milk, ice cream, beef, pork, bacon, hot dogs, sausages, and SPAM are loaded with fat. In most cases, it's the combination of processed foods and fatty animal foods that makes people overweight. Indeed, it is this very combination that leads to overweight, diabetes, and metabolic disorders, including insulin resistance and diabetes.

The Cruel Truth About Insulin Resistance, Weight Gain, and Diabetes

Cells only need a certain amount of blood sugar, or glucose, to function properly. Unfortunately, we are constantly pumping more sugar into the body than is needed. The body attempts to burn the excess sugar, but in order to do that it must force the sugar into the cells where it can be burned as fuel. The body does this by producing more insulin, a substance secreted by the pancreas and primarily responsible for the metabolism of proteins, carbohydrates, and fats. It is a common misconception that insulin only metabolizes carbohydrates; it also metabolizes protein and fat.

Notice that I say "force the sugar into the cells." Actually, cells don't want to be stuffed with more fuel than they can use and thus they limit the amount of fuel they will accept. That means that after a certain point, cells become resistant to the excess sugar, and to the effects of the insulin that is trying to get the sugar into the cells. It's as if the cells have suddenly shut all their doors and shuttered their windows and said, "No more sugar! We're full up!"

Meanwhile, dietary fat also contributes to insulin resistance. Fat coats the exterior of the cells and blocks the insulin receptor sites, the doors and windows through which glucose, the form of sugar that cells can use, passes into the cell. Yes, glucose can still enter the cell, but the body has to produce more insulin in order to force it in.

Fat also infiltrates the cell membrane, where it causes oxidation, which triggers an immune reaction. This creates inflammation within the cell. The inflamed and swollen cell membrane forms a barrier of sorts against the glucose and insulin in the blood, making the cell even more insulin-resistant. In this way, processed foods, excess calories, and fat combine to create extremely stubborn insulin resistance.

Unfortunately, if you keep putting simple, rapidly absorbed carbohydrates into your mouth, your blood-sugar levels will remain high. Now the body has to find a way to overcome its cells' insulin resistance, which is a life-threatening condition. To function optimally, cells need glucose. Without it, cells are at risk of dying. The only thing the body can do to avoid that fate is produce even more insulin.

The additional insulin manages to knock down the doors and penetrate the inflamed and swollen cell membrane, and more and more sugar is stuffed into the cells. But not without a price. High blood sugar, high insulin, and insulin resistance lead to an array of disorders, including overweight, obesity, diabetes, and a condition known as metabolic disorder. As we will see, elevated insulin and glucose also lead to cancer.

Today, there are about 15 million diabetics in the United States alone, about 1.5 million with juvenile diabetes (type 1), and 13.5 million with adult-onset diabetes (type 2). Type 1 diabetes is a condition in which the pancreas does not produce *enough* insulin. In contrast, type 2 diabetes results from the *over*production of insulin that I have just described. A mountain of scientific evidence demonstrates that, by maintaining lean body weight and exercising regularly, many people can prevent diabetes, even if they have a predisposition to the disease.

Very often, people with type 2 diabetes experience intractable insulin resistance. When that happens, medicines are used to force the pancreas to make even more insulin, which then coerces cells into accepting the sugar. Eventually the insulin-producing cells are destroyed, leaving the person unable to produce sufficient amounts of insulin naturally. At that point, they must inject themselves with insulin each day in order to meet their insulin requirements. Without insulin, the body dies.

Long before that happens, however, the morbidly high blood-sugar and insulin levels bring about other dire consequences.

Diabetes: The Slow Destruction of the Body

Adult-onset diabetes is the result of excess calorie consumption, which causes an increase in triglyceride levels. The number-one consequence of diabetes and the resulting inflammation is coronary heart disease. Triglycerides and LDL cholesterol levels rise as excess calories are consumed. Together, the two set inflammation and atherosclerosis raging in arteries throughout the body, so that the limbs, nervous system, and major organs are affected. If the carotid arteries (located in the neck) become inflamed, swollen, and atherosclerotic, the likelihood of stroke is increased. If the arteries that nourish the cells in the legs, feet, arms, and hands become inflamed, the blood supply to the limbs is cut off, and cells and nerves die. When nerves die, you lose feeling in the affected areas, in this case the legs, feet, toes, and fingers. Very often a diabetic does not feel the pain that would alert him or her to the presence of an ingrown toenail or a pebble in the shoe. Infection can easily set in and spread throughout the system, giving rise to a serious and even life-threatening situation.

Eventually, as blood supply is diminished to the feet and legs, gangrene can set in. In extreme cases, there is no other choice but to amputate one or more toes, a foot, or part of the leg. Diabetes is the number-one cause of amputation of limbs.

It's also the number-one cause of blindness, which often occurs when arteries supplying blood to the eyes and retina become inflamed and blocked with atherosclerosis. Cells of the eye atrophy, and scar tissue forms within the eyes. Blood may start to leak out from these tiny vessels. Vision becomes clouded and the retina may become damaged and detached, causing temporary or permanent blindness.

The same process occurs in the kidneys. Here the arteries not only become blocked but many become so thick with inflammation that they are no longer able to expand to allow blood to flow more freely. The effect is not unlike squeezing a hose while water is running through it, causing the pressure to increase. In the case of the body, blood pressure becomes elevated, and pressure is put on the entire arterial system, as well as on the heart.

High glucose and insulin also act as stimulants to cancer cells and tumors. Studies on both humans and animals have shown that tumors are ravenous for glucose. That makes perfect sense, since cancerous cells grow rapidly and require enormous amounts of fuel to maintain their incredible rate of activity. High glucose and insulin may be among the keys to the onset of breast cancer. Writing in the *European Journal of Clinical Nutrition,* Dr. Betsy Stoll, an oncologist at St. Thomas's Hospital in London, stated that in her study "the growth of breast cancer is favored by specific dietary fatty acids, visceral fat accumulation and inadequate physical exercise, all of which are thought to interact in favoring the development of the insulin resistance syndrome" (Stoll 1999).

Also related to overweight, insulin, and cancer is the fact that as weight increases, so, too, do the levels of the reproductive hormones estrogen and testosterone. Researchers have consistently shown that as these hormone levels increase, the risk of breast and prostate cancers goes up sharply as well. Elevated levels of fat, glucose, and insulin may affect certain immune cells and cytokines, which in turn may promote the onset of a variety of cancers (discussed in more detail in chapter 12).

The Easy Road Back to Health

Cheryl and Jim, husband and wife and owners of a restaurant in Nebraska, came to me in the winter of 2000. Cheryl, age 38 at the time of our first meeting, was 50 pounds overweight and diabetic. Her cholesterol level was 206 mg/dL and her triglycerides were 250 mg/dL. Jim, 41, was 60 pounds overweight and also diabetic. He had a cholesterol level of 247 mg/dL and a triglyceride count of 310 mg/dL. Both were used to "the good life," as they put it—too many steaks, cakes, martinis, and late nights. They had one teenage son who was mildly overweight but uninterested in changing his lifestyle. Cheryl and Jim were committed to making a change, however.

Both went on Phase 1 of the Fleming Program, and I followed their progress closely for a year. After nine months on the program, Cheryl weighed 125 and had lost 50 pounds. Her cholesterol was down to 140 mg/dL and her triglycerides, 125 mg/dL. Jim had lost 60 pounds and weighed 150. His cholesterol had fallen to 165 mg/dL, and his triglycerides were 156. Cheryl and Jim had been transformed.

Guaranteeing Weight Loss: Two Simple Principles

Within the dark clouds of this terrible health epidemic lies a simple golden truth that can save us from ourselves: it's all reversible. And to make the news even better, it is not that difficult to restore our health. What we must do to overcome overweight, diabetes, and most of the other illnesses that accompany these killers is to reduce caloric intake and increase exercise.

By significantly reducing the number of calories you consume you can:

- Cause weight loss until you reach your goal for a normal, healthy weight.
- Dramatically reduce blood sugar to restore normal blood-sugar levels.
- Dramatically lower insulin levels to restore normal insulin levels.
- Reduce inflammation throughout your body and improve your immune system.
- Burn more fat effortlessly and continually.
- Restore insulin sensitivity.
- Overcome type 2 diabetes.
- If you have type 1 diabetes, you can lower your insulin requirements and prevent a wide array of diabetes-related illnesses, including heart disease, kidney disorders, loss of vision, claudication, and neuropathy.
- Reduce blood pressure.
- Improve and restore circulation throughout your body, particularly in your limbs, toes, fingers, and nerve fibers.
- Take the stress off your heart and vascular system.
- Reduce your risk of cancer and other serious illnesses.

- Improve sleep and energy levels.
- Dramatically improve your skin and overall appearance.
- Improve sexual potency and function.

The Fleming Program can help you achieve all of these goals easily and quickly. Allow me to explain first how weight loss is accomplished and then show you how it can be done relatively easily, and relatively quickly. In order to lose weight, you have to understand and practice two simple principles.

The First Simple Principle of Weight Loss

The first principle is the easy math of weight loss. (Don't panic—it's fun!) It takes about 10 calories to maintain a pound of your current weight, so if you weigh 200 pounds you need 2,000 calories a day to stay at that weight. That, by the way, is a lot of food, and a lot of calories. If you were to consume, say, 1,500 calories a day (still a good-size diet), you'd be getting enough calories to support a weight of only 150 pounds. Let's say that you weigh 150 pounds, but you really want to weigh 120. All you have to do is drop your calorie consumption down to 1,200 calories per day—the level most nutritionists regard as a normal amount of food per day for the average person.

If you cut out 350 to 500 calories a day, you will lose about a pound a week. (Since water is trapped in fat tissue, your weight loss may be more than a pound per week.) If you eat the standard Western diet of meat, processed foods, and sugar, you can easily eliminate 350 to 500 calories a day and not even miss that food. Most overweight people can easily lose 50 pounds a year if they want to and not even feel deprived.

But by far the best and easiest way to shed pounds is to eat a diet that's low in calories and rich in nutrition and fiber. Such a diet will cause healthful weight loss while it improves your overall health.

The Second Simple Principle of Weight Loss

The second principle of weight loss is maintaining low glucose and insulin levels by eating whole, unprocessed vegetables, beans, grains, and fruit. Whole, unprocessed foods contain what are called complex carbohydrates, as opposed to simple sugars. And when it comes to weight loss and healthy insulin levels, this makes all the difference in the world. Complex carbohydrates are long chains of sugars that are bound up in a fiber. The sugars are essentially tied up within the strands of this ropelike fiber. In order for these sugars to be released, digestive enzymes and your small intestine must work together to break down the fiber and separate the sugars from the chemical bonds that hold them within their chains. This requires hours of work, which is the reason why complex carbohydrates found in vegetables, beans, and whole grains provide many hours of energy. If you eat, say, a bowl of oatmeal or brown rice or squash, the sugars will be released into your bloodstream over a matter of several hours. A whole food at breakfast will give you lots of energy and endurance until lunch. A whole food at lunch will give you enduring energy until dinner, and a dinner of whole, unprocessed foods will give you energy until bedtime, and right on through to the next morning.

These enduring waves of energy are long arcs, rather than a spike that rises quickly and falls off just as quickly. Sugar and other processed foods give your body that glucose and insulin spike, whereas whole, unprocessed nutritious foods provide the long energy arc.

As long as you eat whole, unprocessed plant foods and avoid processed foods you will maintain a steady flow of blood glucose and relatively low insulin levels. When glucose and insulin are low, you will burn a fuel mixture of about 50 percent glucose and 50 percent fat. In effect, moderate glucose levels force you to burn fat as a supplemental fuel source. That means you are consuming your fat reserves even when you are not exercising, which means you are losing weight while sitting or even lying down.

Halfway Measures Fail

One of the main reasons why people have trouble losing weight today is that they believe they can shed pounds by eating less of the same foods they are already eating. But this is impossible. The standard Western diet is made up almost entirely of processed and high-fat foods. That's why we're overweight and sick. *You cannot eat a smaller amount of the foods that caused your health problem and expect to restore your health.* This is like pouring a quart of gasoline on a fire, instead of a gallon, and expecting the fire to go out. These foods are too rich in calories, too pro-inflammatory, and too detrimental to health. People who fool themselves into thinking they can "eat around" the "problem foods" are only fooling themselves.

If you are overweight, you are either already ill, or at a very high risk of becoming ill. You know in your heart that significant change is needed. You probably know that either you must bring about that change, or it will be brought about for you as a result of a medical emergency. The Fleming Program is an alternative to a great deal of suffering.

The best way to cut out calories and include immune system–boosting, health-promoting foods is to make a complete break with the old ways of eating. Change the food entirely and give your body what it really needs. The people who adopt my program find it easy to adhere to the recommendations because they are clear, decisive, and unambiguous. That means that you will not have to suffer the same temptation as those who eat "just a little bread, or "just a small amount of cheese," or "just one or two hamburgers." Those foods are gone—at least until you have achieved your goals for Phase 1. By the time you get to Phase 2, you'll have much greater freedom to enjoy some of the old foods, but in much smaller quantities. By that time, however, you will have experienced what it is like to be lean, healthy, full of energy, clear of eye, and sharp of mind. I'm betting that at that point you will know your limits. You'll also know what to eat if you regain a pound or two or suffer unwanted symptoms.

A Cheney-like Case History

Ironically, I was recently confronted with a patient whose condition resembles that of the vice president's in many details. In January 2001, a 63-year-old college professor from Washington, D.C., came to see me with severe angina pain, a long history of overweight and heart disease, and very few medical options left.

Twenty-two years earlier, in the fall of 1979, he began experiencing angina pain and later that year suffered his first heart attack, after which he underwent coronary bypass surgery. Eight years later he had another heart attack and underwent a balloon angioplasty. Between 1990 and 1994 he had numerous angioplasties. In 1995 he had a supporting device called a tubular stent implanted in one of his coronary arteries. The stent collapsed three weeks later. In order to open the artery and prevent another heart attack, the professor underwent a second bypass operation. At that point he began a widely known low-fat vegetarian diet. He lost about 10 pounds but continued to suffer angina pain after minimal exertion. He could not walk up a single flight of stairs without intense angina pain, which not only stopped him in his tracks but also left him in terror of sudden death.

Five years later, in December 2000, angiograms showed that all three of his major coronary arteries were significantly occluded, despite the two bypass operations, the stent, and several angioplasties. One of his main coronary arteries was blocked; another was 70 percent closed. He was surviving only because he had extensive collateral, or secondary, circulation to the heart muscle. He suffered from severe angina pain after only minor exertion. He had regained 40 pounds, so he was still 50 pounds overweight. Like Vice President Cheney, he was clinging to life by a very thin thread.

His physicians suggested that he explore four possible options: find another self-help program that would give better results; try laser surgery to open his coronary arteries; get a heart transplant; or make out his will. Of those four, three were useless. Laser surgery would not increase the blood flow to his heart; he was not a viable candidate for a heart transplant; and his will was already taken care of. That left him with option number one, which eventually led him to me.

I did a complete workup of him and discovered that the combination of medication and his low-fat diet had lowered his cholesterol significantly—his total cholesterol was a very healthy 110. Obviously, lowering his cholesterol was not the single answer. But other important risk factors were in the danger zones, including his weight.

I explained my approach to him and placed him on the Phase 1 program: the Phase 1 diet, exercise, and supplements. I also changed his medication significantly and took him off fish oil supplement he was taking. Fish oil is a form of fat, and it very likely was reducing the oxygen-carrying capacity of his blood. He followed my treatment program to the letter. Two months later, he had lost 20 pounds and was able to walk for three miles without any angina. During the next two months he lost

> ### REVERSING HEART DISEASE ON THE FLEMING PROGRAM: STEP 3
>
> **Normalize your weight by cutting at least 500 calories per day from your diet. This is easily accomplished by adopting the Fleming Phase 1 diet. Once you've achieved your ideal weight, maintain it with Phase 2 of the Fleming Program.**
>
> *

another 20 pounds. At the same time, his overall health, blood values, and fitness improved dramatically. Soon, he was able to ride an exercise bicycle daily. His energy had increased considerably and he had no signs of angina. Other tests showed an improved blood flow to his heart. Today, he has lost all the excess weight. He is lean, his numbers are all within normal ranges, and he reports that he feels better than he has in more than 20 years.

How Exercise Improves Health

WE'VE KNOWN FOR A LONG TIME THAT regular exercise is associated with low rates of heart disease and heart attacks. What we didn't fully understand is the mechanisms of exercise's protective benefits. Exercise improves many factors within the blood, including raising HDL levels. It also strengthens the heart muscle. Still, those benefits alone do not explain why even small amounts of exercise significantly improve heart health. New research is now throwing light on why exercise is so protective: exercise reduces inflammation throughout the body, including in the arteries. Since inflammation is the underlying cause of heart disease, exercise is essential medicine for the heart.

Scientists have recently been focusing on an element in the blood, C-reactive protein (C-RP), which reveals how much inflammation is occurring in the body. A study done at Emory University in Atlanta examined the exercise patterns of 3,638 healthy men and women, all 40 and older, and found that those who engaged in the lowest amounts of physical activity each month, three exercise sessions or less, had the highest levels of C-RP, indicating the highest levels of inflammation. Those who engaged in moderate physical activity, 4 to 21 times per month, had significantly lower levels of C-RP, and those who exercised frequently, 22 times per month or more, had the lowest levels of C-RP, indicating the lowest levels of inflammation.

If you walk five or six times per week for at least 30 minutes, you will exercise 20 to 24 times a month. The effect of that much exercise will mean significantly lower C-RP levels and inflammation, including in your arteries. With less inflammation comes a much lower risk of heart attack.

A study done by Dr. Michael J. LaMonte of the University of Utah in Salt Lake turned up similar findings. LaMonte and his colleagues compared the effects of fitness on C-RP blood levels in 135 women representing a variety of racial backgrounds. Rather than simply asking the women how much they exercised each month, LaMonte had each woman walk on a treadmill until she was too fatigued to continue and then categorized each woman's fitness level. Once he determined a woman's actual fitness, he measured her C-RP level. Like the Emory study, LaMonte found that the least-fit women had the highest levels of C-RP, and thus the highest levels of inflammation. Conversely, those who were most physically fit had the lowest levels of C-RP and the lowest inflammation. LaMonte concluded that "the health benefits from enhanced fitness may have an anti-inflammatory mechanism" (LaMonte 2002).

A study done collaboratively by the Cooper Institute of Aerobics Research in Dallas, Texas, and the Centers for Disease Control (*Journal of American Medicine*, November 1989), involving some 14,000 participants, confirmed these findings.

High Blood Pressure and Inflammation

Not surprisingly, elevated C-RP levels are also associated with higher risk of high blood pressure (Abramson, Weintraub, et al. 2002). High blood pressure is a major risk factor for heart attack and stroke. That inflammation increases a person's risk of hypertension only stands to reason, since one of the underlying causes of hypertension is the inability of arteries to expand. When the heart beats faster, more blood is pumped throughout the system. In order to accommodate that increase in blood supply, the arteries must expand.

However, arteries that are inflamed and swollen are unable to expand. When more blood attempts to flow through a narrow vessel, blood pressure naturally increases. The increase in blood pressure typically seen with aging was the basis for increasing the "normal" range for blood pressure above 120/80 mm (millimeters of mercury). However, this increase in blood pressure is not a good thing and has resulted in many people being told their blood pressure is all right. Having a little increase in blood pressure is like being a little pregnant: You either are or you aren't.

This increased pressure places enormous stress on the walls of the artery, causing tiny fissures to appear. These bring about even greater inflammation and atherosclerosis, the underlying cause of most heart attacks and strokes. But even before either of those events occurs, there are numerous other side effects that can dramatically alter your life. High blood pressure is a major cause of blindness, kidney disorders, and sexual dysfunction.

Scientists have known for decades that blood pressure can be reduced through exercise and weight loss. Both reduce inflammation, which can restore health to blood vessels.

Exercise, Fibrinogen, and Blood Clots

Exercise affects other blood factors that increase the risk of heart attacks. A British study of more than 3,800 men, published in the April 2002 issue of *Circulation*, the journal of the American Heart Association (Wannamethee et al. 2002) showed that men between the ages of 60 and 79 who exercised regularly had lower levels not only of C-RP but also of fibrinogen, a blood protein that increases the tendency of the blood to form clots. Blood clots are an underlying cause of most heart attacks. By reducing the blood's tendency to clot, exercise offers major protection against heart attack.

The British researchers also found that the blood of men who exercised regularly was far less viscous, which meant that it was better able to circulate to cells and organs throughout the body, including the heart.

Go Slow and Still Benefit

You do not have to walk fast, or particularly far, to gain enormous benefits from walking. A study published in the *Journal of the American Medical As-*

sociation (JAMA) found that women who walked at a leisurely pace of about three miles per hour were far less likely to suffer from heart disease than women who did not walk at all. The scientists divided a population of women into four groups: one group did not walk at all; one group did a 20-minute mile; another did a 15-minute mile; and a third walked a 12-minute mile. All the women who walked, no matter what their speed, saw their HDL levels increase 6 percent. According to J. J. Duncan, a Cooper Institute researcher and the lead author of the study, "That increase in HDL translates into an 18 percent drop in heart disease risk" (Duncan 1991). And that's purely from taking a stroll a few times per week.

Exercise, Diabetes, Insulin, and Inflammation

People who do not exercise are far more likely to be overweight and insulin-resistant. Insulin resistance leads to increased inflammation, heart disease, diabetes, and even cancer. Exercise burns excess carbohydrates, increases insulin sensitivity, and lowers both glucose and insulin levels. In the process, exercise helps to prevent adult-onset, or type 2, diabetes. When you couple exercise with a diet low in fat and calories, the protective effects are even more powerful.

The latest study to demonstrate the power of exercise and diet to prevent diabetes is the Diabetes Prevention Program, a large clinical trial involving more than 3,000 people, undertaken by the National Institute of Diabetes and Digestive and Kidney Diseases (*New England Journal of Medicine,* 2002). The study showed that people most at risk for contracting adult-onset diabetes, those with chronically high insulin levels, could protect themselves from the illness by exercising 30 minutes a day—a simple walk is enough—and by consuming fewer calories and less fat and processed foods. The researchers found that exercise and diet were nearly twice as effective at preventing the illness as any drug treatments.

Exercise, Immune-System Boosting, and Cancer

Moderate exercise—that 30-minute walk done at a comfortable pace—is enough to make your immune cells stronger and more numerous. This is especially the case for the immune system's primary defender against cancer, the natural killer (NK) cells. The job of NK cells is to target cancer cells, tumors and destroy them. With regular, moderate exercise, NK cells become more numerous in the bloodstream and more aggressive, especially when they locate a cancer cell or tumor. Researchers have found that this effect even occurs in elderly women who take up some form of regular, gentle exercise.

Exercise has the same effect on all classes of immune cells, including macrophages, which replicate more rapidly and become more alert and aggressive in people who exercise regularly. They also become far more active where there is inflammation, including in the arteries. It's possible that exercise may make macrophages more effective at cleaning up the areas in the body where inflammation is chronic.

Research has consistently shown that exercise protects women against breast cancer. Women whose lifestyles are active, and who burn a lot of calories each day, have breast cancer rates that are 10 to 20 percent below the average. On the other hand, sedentary women have a breast cancer rate that is 30 percent above the average, according to a study done jointly by the National Cancer Institute and the Shanghai Cancer Institute in China (Zheng 1993).

One study found that women who exercised an average of 48 minutes a week were less likely to develop breast cancer than those who did not exercise at all. Those women who exercised about four hours per week had the lowest rates.

The data consistently point to the same conclusion: by reducing inflammation, exercise addresses the fundamental causes of many life-threatening illnesses.

And You May Live Longer, Too

All of which explains why exercise may help you live longer. Several studies have shown that people who exercise regularly live longer than those who do not. A study published in the *New England Journal of Medicine* reported that men between the ages of 45 and 54 who adopt a vigorous exercise program live, on average, 10 months longer than those who remain sedentary (Paffenbarger 1993).

Perhaps the most persuasive of these reports was published in the *Journal of the American Medical Association*. In that study, done by the Cooper In-

...pics Research in Dallas, researchers determined the fitness
...tterns of 13,344 men and women and then followed them for
...e scientists divided the study participants into five groups, from
...st fit. The least fit did no exercise at all; the second group only
...ext two groups participated in various sports or physical fitness
...he fifth group was comprised of long-distance runners, including
marathoners.

The scientists found that the least-fit people—those who did no exercise at all—had the highest death rate within the eight-year period. That was expected. What they didn't expect, however, was that the greatest difference in mortality rates was between the least fit and the next category up, the group of people who merely walked four or five times a week. The four groups that did any exercise—the walkers and the athletes—had relatively similar death rates. The death rate among the least fit was three times that of the walkers. A relatively small amount of exercise, namely walking, created the biggest difference in health and longevity (Blair 1989).

"Even modest amounts of exercise can substantially reduce a person's chances of dying" of heart disease, cancer, and other illnesses, it was reported in the November 3, 1989, *New York Times*. "This is a hopeful message, an important message for the American people to understand," Dr. Carl Caspersen of the Centers for Disease Control told the *Times*. "You don't have to be a marathoner. In fact, you get much more benefit out of being just a bit more active. For example, going from being sedentary to walking briskly for a half hour several days a week can drop your risk dramatically."

Add to this the fact that exercise strengthens bones and can prevent osteoporosis, a major cause of disability and death among the elderly, and we begin to see why this behavior is so absolutely essential. As one researcher told *Time* magazine: "Regular physical activity is probably as close to a magic bullet as we will [see] in modern medicine."

It's Easier to Eat Healing Foods If You Exercise

Here's a remarkable fact about exercise that people experience, but often fail to realize: People who exercise prefer more healthful foods naturally. This is not just my personal observation but a well-supported scientific statement.

Studies consistently show that people who regularly exercise are far more likely to maintain a healthy diet, lose weight, and keep the weight off, than those who diet but do not exercise. Why is this so? Because exercise makes us crave carbohydrate-rich foods, which, if you choose the right ones, will cause rapid and ongoing weight loss. They will also boost your health in every other way. Here's what happens.

Your body is able to store a lot of calories as fat. A lean person stores about 100,000 calories as fat in their tissues, and an overweight person has two to three times that amount. By contrast, our capacity to store carbohydrates is limited to about 1,500 calories, which we store primarily in the muscles and liver.

Your fuel mix tends to be 50 percent carbohydrates and 50 percent fat. Since you have a lot more fat than carbohydrates stored in your tissues, your carb supply is going to be the first to empty, especially if you exercise. Exercise causes muscles to work. Since carbs are stored in the muscles, they are burned rapidly, leaving a carbohydrate deficit in the body.

Your brain prefers carbohydrates as its primary fuel source. When your carbohydrate fuel supply drops, the brain recognizes the deficit and immediately triggers cravings for carbohydrate-rich foods. Once that craving is created, you should choose whole, unprocessed plant foods, as opposed to processed fare.

You will recall from the previous chapter that plant foods contain complex carbohydrates that are slowly absorbed. These foods are low in calories and thus promote weight loss. Good sources of these slow-burning, complex carbs are brown rice, oatmeal, millet, and other grains, as well as pulpy vegetables such as beans, squash, and sweet potatoes. These foods are so low in calories that eating them will not lead to excess weight. You will lose weight, even as you eat all the food your body desires.

In essence, exercise makes it easier for you to stay on a healthy diet, because it triggers cravings for plant foods, which provide your brain with its preferred fuel.

Research has consistently confirmed this process. Scientists divided a population of rats into two groups, one that was made to exercise and the other that was allowed to live a sedentary lifestyle. The rats were given their choice of two food supplies, one high in fat, and the other low in fat and high in carbohydrates. The rats that exercised consistently chose the low-fat, high-carb food supply, while the sedentary rats consistently chose the high-fat regimen (Gerardo-Gettens 1991).

The same effects occur in humans. A study by researchers at Stanford University (Wood et al. 1985) followed a group of middle-aged men who maintained a daily running regime for two years. The scientists gave the runners no nutritional advice, but closely monitored their dietary choices. The researchers made a couple of interesting findings. First, the appetites of the men increased, as did their overall food intake. Second, their consumption of carbohydrate-rich foods increased. Third, all the runners lost weight, even though their appetites and the amount of food they ate increased.

This study was reproduced by E. J. Simoes and his colleagues, who found that the more people—both men and women—exercise, the more carbohydrate-rich foods they eat (Simoes 1995). Other studies have since supported this finding.

These results help to explain why people who exercise tend to lose weight and keep it off. Exercise causes your body to burn more calories. It also strengthens and builds existing muscles. Muscle is very active tissue. Unlike fat cells, which are very inactive, muscle tissue is constantly burning calories. The bigger your muscles, the more calories you burn. Also, exercise speeds up metabolism, which causes your system to burn more calories even while you are resting.

All of these reasons add up to more calorie burning and weight loss. But perhaps the most intriguing reason is the last one: the tendency of exercise to cause changes in your diet—healthful, weight-reducing changes—that encourage rapid, healthful, and significant weight loss. It's also exercise that keeps weight off after you've lost it.

Meanwhile, It Makes You Feel Better About Being You

Very few activities can boost your self-esteem like exercise, primarily because it triggers positive changes in brain chemistry. Studies have shown that after 20 minutes of moderately intense exercise, you can experience a significant decrease in anxiety and an elevation of mood and optimism. With continued exercise, you can even lift off into mild states of euphoria, thanks to the brain's increase in production of beta endorphins. These morphine-like compounds create feelings of well-being and the "natural high" that is often mentioned by people who exercise regularly.

Such changes explain why exercise has been shown to reduce and even, for some, eliminate depression. The July 1990 issue of *Postgraduate Medicine* reported a study that examined the effects of regular exercise on people who suffered from chronic depression and anxiety. The researchers found that those who exercised daily experienced a significant diminution of negative mood states, along with an elevation in feelings of optimism and well-being. The study participants also reported that their ability to deal with stress improved dramatically so that stressful situations did not result in either depression or intense or anxious feelings. The participants stated that after they began exercising regularly, they did not indulge in negative thinking or excessive self-criticism as they had done before they began their exercise regimen. Instead, they found themselves feeling far healthier, emotionally balanced, optimistic, and more positive about their lives.

The Key to Becoming Your Best Self

Ron was a 67-year-old retired college professor and high school administrator who came to me in the fall of 2000 with chronic chest pain, high blood pressure, and obesity. He was six feet tall and weighed 220, which meant that he was about 50 pounds overweight. Until I did a SPECT test of his heart, Ron didn't know that he had also suffered a mild heart attack, which had caused part of his heart muscle to die.

"It must have been one of those times when I thought I had gas," Ron later said laughing. "I never knew it. I did have chest pain pretty regularly, but it never got so bad that I thought I was having a heart attack."

I put Ron on the Phase 1 diet and exercise program. Not only did he adhere to the diet perfectly, but he routinely walked two miles a day, and often as many as four. Within a year he lost 50 pounds and was no longer suffering from angina and high blood pressure. Remarkably, part of his heart tissue that had not been getting sufficient oxygen but was still alive recovered and started working normally. Of course, the tissue that had died from his heart attack could not be restored, but because of the increased blood flow, his heart was working far better than it had in years.

For me, Ron's case is especially interesting because he had a reason to get well that went beyond simple survival. Ron was a pilot and he absolutely loved to fly. When his heart disease was diagnosed, his pilot's license was revoked. Getting back his license became a powerful motivation to regain his health.

"Ever since I was a kid, I loved airplanes," Ron recalled. "Whenever I was flying, I would say to myself, 'My God, what joy.'" In fact, he never fully understood why he hadn't become a commercial pilot. He served in the Air Force during the Korean War, but not as a pilot. After he was discharged, he went back to college. "I studied math and science on the G.I. bill," Ron continued. "And after college, I went on to graduate school, but my love of flying never faded away. One day, after I was out of graduate school, I decided to learn to fly. I loved it the minute I got into the cockpit. I had known I would. I got my pilot's license. And from that time on, I never could figure out why I hadn't done it for a living."

But when clear signs of heart disease emerged, Ron was forced to undergo a rigorous physical, which revealed his coronary heart disease. "They gave me a physical and I flunked it," Ron remembered. "And from that day on, I realized that I had to get my health back because I wanted to fly so badly."

On the Phase 1 program, Ron discovered another thing he loved, though he didn't know it until he began the diet. "I discovered that I love vegetables and fruit," he said recently. "My parents were livestock farmers, and we grew up on meat and potatoes. But once I started this diet, I found that I really enjoy all the vegetables and fruit. I love sweet potatoes and squash, broccoli, onions, cauliflower, salads, peppers, and radishes. I really enjoy cherries, and blueberries, and pineapple, and peaches. A lot of the time, I mix salad greens and tomatoes and fruit and I whip up a delicious salad. After I got on to Phase 2, I just never stopped eating mostly vegetables and fruit. And now, I've learned how to make bread, so I make a big bowl of vegetable soup and eat it with salad and bread. Today, I eat a piece of steak maybe once a month. I eat fish, too. But once I got on the Phase 1 program, I never stopped making vegetables and fruit the center of my diet. That's how I lost so much weight. I just kept eating the vegetables and fruit and kept losing weight."

The other thing that he discovered he loved when he began the Fleming Program was golf. "I took up golf because it's a game that I thought I would enjoy and it's good for you. You're outdoors, and of course you're doing a lot of walking. I got bitten by the bug, so to speak. I'm retired, so I play about five times a week. I read someplace recently that eighteen holes of golf is, on average, about four miles of walking. So it's a pretty good workout."

Today, Ron is in his best physical condition of the past 30 years. And needless to say, he's flying again.

Ron's story illustrates the importance of having something you enjoy doing as an incentive to start a diet and exercise program. Clearly, it's not enough for people to know the physical, mental, and emotional benefits of exercise. Most people change their lives because they need to be healthy in order to do something that they truly enjoy doing. In other words, you need to remember the man or woman inside of you who longed to be good at a certain game, or who dreamed of becoming a black belt in karate, or a good dancer or tennis player, or to function at your best at your job.

I know a man who always loved baseball, but thought the game was gone from his life after he reached the age of 30. When he was 41, he discovered a 40-and-over baseball league and decided to give it a try. His old love of the game came roaring back, and pretty soon he wanted to be a good player again. So he started working out a couple of times a week, walked every day, and lost 20 pounds. Then he decided to go to one of those dream baseball vacations where you get to play with retired big league ballplayers. So he started working out a little more to get into shape. They play baseball all day long at those camps and this man wanted to be in good shape so that he could perform at his best. As it turned out, the camp was both fun and inspirational, in part because many of the ex–big-leaguers were in great shape and could still play ball better than all the amateurs put together. The retired big-leaguers served as models for aging. After my friend came back home, he vowed to stay in shape and continue to play baseball every summer until he was too old to see the ball. To this day, he continues to be in excellent health and fitness—all for his love of the game. This is very common. I know tennis players and golfers in their fifties who love their respective sports so much that they wouldn't dream of letting themselves get out of shape because it would diminish their fun.

Not long ago, I read an article about the talented British golfer Colin Montgomery, who lost 40 or 50 pounds in a short period of time. When asked what motivated him to take off all those pounds, Montgomery replied that he simply didn't want to be fat anymore—didn't want to see himself as fat. When I read that article, I realized that Colin Montgomery had visualized his best self, the part of him that was lean and fit and was able to utilize his remarkable talents. Being overweight didn't allow him to do that. When he saw the heroic image of himself in his mind's eye, he changed his way of eating and began exercising vigorously. And it wasn't long before he lost a great deal of weight.

The best version of you is not overweight, nor is it a you who is a glutton for unhealthy food. The best version of you eats well and is lean, fit, and vigorous, right into old age. In fact, old age is not "old" when you are fit and healthy, because you face fewer limitations than when you are overweight and unhealthy. The great cancer researcher Dr. Ernst Wynder said, "Die young, as late in life as possible."

Let me tell you something about exercise that is very rarely written about or spoken of, but is widely known by people who do it every day: exercise strengthens your will and makes you realize that virtually anything is possible for you! Once you start exercising daily, you feel yourself getting stronger and more effective in life. In a strange and almost miraculous way, you start to realize that you can use your creative powers to create the life you want to live.

That's one of the reasons why I say that the first step in becoming the best version of yourself is to exercise daily. Couple that with the Fleming Program diet and you can experience abundant energy and the emergence of the attractive and beautiful you.

The Fleming Exercise Program

First Things First

Before you start exercising, you must do two things. First, get a thorough physical from your doctor, including an electrocardiogram and a stress test on a treadmill to make sure that any exercise regimen that you start will not be harmful. Ask your doctor how much exercise is wise for you to undertake, and if there are any restrictions on your regimen. Start out slow. The exercise component of Phase 1 is essentially a walking program, nothing more, but it's enough to improve your fitness and cardiovascular health. When your overall condition is stronger, you can include a sport or some other more vigorous activity.

Second, you must change your way of eating. Don't adopt an exercise program without adopting the Phase 1 diet. If you exercise but continue to eat a high-fat, high-calorie diet, the inflammatory processes will continue and the atherosclerotic plaque will grow, even as you exercise. The exercise will place greater demands on your heart for oxygen, but your arteries will not be able to provide the blood and oxygen the heart needs. That combination can be very dangerous. Adopt the Fleming Phase 1 diet and then start the moderate exercise regimen.

Exercise in Phase 1

Two thirds of Americans get little or no exercise, which helps to explain why two thirds of Americans are overweight. What's really remarkable is that it takes so little effort to take a daily walk. Some people complain that they don't have enough time, but I don't buy that excuse. You can walk for 30 minutes during your lunch hour, or take three 10-minute walks a day—one in the morning, one in the afternoon, and one in the evening.

Many researchers, and I am among them, believe that if people walked 30 minutes a day, we could reduce the incidence of most chronic diseases—including heart disease, diabetes, and cancer—by 30 to 50 percent.

Here's what I recommend. If you are not exercising at all, begin by taking three walks a week. Either make each walk at least 30 minutes long, or take three 10-minute walks a day. Once you get in the habit of doing three days a week and you find that your fitness level is improving, graduate to a 30-minute walk five or six days a week. That's optimal on Phase 1.

Do not overdo it, either with speed or duration. Walk at a pace that allows you to speak to a friend or cowalker without losing your breath. If you haven't exercised and are just starting out on your exercise program, begin by strolling. At the outset, limit your distance to under two miles. Most of all, enjoy your walk. Don't push it. Remember that at the outset, duration and distance are much more important than speed.

You may want to use a treadmill—one of the greatest investments you can make in your health. A treadmill allows you to walk every day, at a variety of speeds, no matter what the weather or the terrain. Set up a treadmill in a room where you can watch television while you walk, or where you can listen to music. Walk at a pace that is enjoyable and not overly strenuous. Remember, distance matters more than speed. But even when considering how far to walk, don't overdo it. Start out at under two miles. Treadmills are especially good for seniors or for people with leg or knee injuries. The soft padded treadmill absorbs shock and softens the impact on your feet and legs.

That's all you have to do on Phase 1. It's easy. It's cheap. And it's safe. Once you have achieved your Phase 1 goals, then graduate to the Phase 2 exercise program.

Exercise in Phase 2

Phase 2 includes a daily 30-minute walk, taken at a brisk pace, five to six days a week, and some other exercise activity. For the walk, do 10 minutes of gentle stretching exercises before and after your walk. Then you'll add a sport or activity that you enjoy, which you will engage in at least twice, and preferably three or four times, a week. Here are my recommendations for possible activities that you can include as part of your exercise regimen.

1. *Walk on a treadmill.* A treadmill on which you can change the speed and elevation can offer a more vigorous, challenging workout in Phase 2, as you work your way up to longer distances and daily exercise. There's no better machine for getting a safe and effective workout and promoting your health.

2. *Golf.* Golf is good workout for those who are willing to forgo the gas-driven cart and instead use a hand-cart to transport their clubs to the 9 or 18 holes. Lots of walking, lots of fun (not to mention frustration!), and lots of fresh air. If you enjoy golf, play often and walk the course. The golfers I have met are often very relaxed people. They love the game. Contrary to what you might expect, they also say that the game gives them a remarkable degree of peace. Take up the game and let it change both your health and outlook on life.

3. *Yoga.* Yoga is a gentle, meditative form of exercise that stretches and strengthens muscles, increases range of motion, improves circulation, and significantly enhances the quality of life. It can be done by just about anyone. Yoga classes are offered in practically every town and city in the United States, as well as Europe and Asia. It's easy and cheap and can make a world of difference in your health.

5. *Dancing.* Ballroom, tango, swing, square dancing, and aerobic dancing are all good workouts. Dancing requires tremendous coordination and

balance. Most forms of dancing are also highly aerobic, fun,
and romantic. Classes are provided in just about every town
or city. Check your Yellow
Pages and local newspapers.

6. *Martial arts.* Tai chi chaun is a
dancelike form of martial art
that can be done by people of
all ages. It requires slow, delib-
erate movements that keep
you focused and centered in
your body and help develop

REVERSING HEART DISEASE ON
THE FLEMING PROGRAM:
STEP 4

Walk for a minimum of 30 minutes
a day, at least three days a week,
and preferably five or six days a
week. When your condition improves, increase your distance and
adopt physical activities that you
enjoy and will do consistently.

coordination and muscle strength. Tai chi, as it is often called, is great for
senior citizens who want to improve their balance, coordination, and
strength. It will not tax your heart excessively, but will give you a nice
workout.

Other forms of martial arts, such as karate, aikido, and tai kwan do,
are far more vigorous and require considerably more effort. They provide
a wonderful workout, but they are only for those who are in good physical condition or have entered the Phase 2 program. See your Yellow
Pages or newspaper for classes.

7. *Gyms and health clubs.* Join a gym or health club or the YMCA or
YWCA, if there is one in your city. Most health clubs have knowledge-
able people who can direct you to the right form of exercise for your
health and fitness level. Check your Yellow Pages or newspaper for a
health club near you.

8. *Stationary bicycle.* A stationary bicycle is a wonderful exercise machine
that provides a highly aerobic form of exercise. For those in good shape,
or on Phase 2, a stationary bicycle will strengthen the legs, heart, and circulation. Most bikes allow you to adjust the rate of difficulty, allowing
you to simulate flat terrain or hills. Start out on the flat terrain; don't
overdo it or stress yourself beyond your capacity. A stationary bike, like a
treadmill, can be a fun and practical way to exercise in your home every
day of the year.

The Two Most Important Rules for Exercise:
Fun and Consistency

The key to exercise is to enjoy yourself. Don't strain yourself or push yourself beyond your limits. Consistency is more important than intensity. Our goal is health and longevity, not perfection. Walk, play a game, or engage in some form of physical activity for the fun of it. The rewards of exercise flow to those who walk or play a game for the pure enjoyment—and experience that enjoyment every day!

Homocysteine and Antioxidants

WHEN RUSSELL CAME TO SEE ME IN THE fall of 2001, he was a 38-year-old competitive bodybuilder who was suffering from periodic chest pain, low energy, and bouts of weakness, a common symptom of significant heart disease. His father had died of a heart attack at the age of 65. His mother, who was still alive, had angina pectoris. Like many bodybuilders, Russell believed that he had to follow a high-protein diet in order to build and sustain muscle mass. Consequently, he ate a lot of animal foods, including steak, hamburgers, eggs, and pork, as well as the dairy products cheese and milk. Daily, he drank a high-protein drink, composed mostly of dairy or soy proteins. He also avoided plant foods as much as possible on the belief that they would cause unwanted weight gain. He did have a sweet tooth, however. "I love chocolate, candy, and even fruit," he told me. "Can't stay away from sweets."

I ran a series of blood tests and then did a SPECT test on his heart. Sure enough, owing to excessive inflammation, his heart was not getting sufficient oxygen, which was the reason he had periodic chest pain. He also had an array of markers for heart disease. His blood cholesterol level was 226 mg/dL, which was dangerously high. At 15 μmol/dL, his homocysteine level was also high ("μmol" stands for "micromole," one millionth of a mole, which is an international unit of chemical measurement). And his C-reactive protein level was at 2.1 mg/dL, also high. The whole picture added up to high inflammation and coronary artery disease, which the SPECT test confirmed. Russell was right to be worried. He was following in the footsteps of his father, only his heart attack would probably come at a younger age.

"I have nothing against bodybuilding, Russell, but your pursuit of the perfect physique is killing you," I said.

"How? Why?" he said, baffled.

"The diet you're using to boost muscle mass is creating inflammation throughout your system, especially in the arteries that lead to your heart," I told him. "That inflammation is creating plaques that are obstructing the blood flow to your heart and causing pain. If you don't change your way of eating, eventually those plaques will erupt and cause a heart attack."

"What's wrong with my diet?" Russell asked.

"The excessive amounts of protein are causing certain chemicals in your blood to rise to toxic levels," I said. "They're inflaming and injuring your arteries and causing the cholesterol plaques to get bigger. Right now, they're cutting off some of the blood to your heart. If you continue doing what you're doing, one or another of those plaques will erupt and cause a heart attack or stroke, depending on what organ the artery goes to, your heart or your brain.

"In addition, the sugar you're eating is raising your blood sugar and insulin levels," I continued. "High insulin also causes inflammation, which contributes to your heart condition.

"Your immune system is trying to stop this process," I said. "But the quantity of those poisonous chemicals is too high for your immune system to deal with. At the same time, you don't feed your body the nutrients that your immune system needs to be strong and win the battle with these poisons. Basically, you've got too many bad guys and not enough good guys. We've got to change that if you want to avoid a heart attack. Are you willing to change your way of eating?" I asked him.

"Yes," he said, obviously a bit shocked. "I feel lousy. Somehow I knew I was on the edge."

I placed Russell on my Phase 1 diet. Once the Phase 1 goals were met, I put him on my Phase 2 program. Ten months after our initial visit, Russell's cholesterol level had fallen to 180 mg/dL and his triglycerides, homocysteine, and C-RP levels were well into the normal ranges. He had no chest pain and was off all medication. But perhaps more important, at least from Russell's point of view, was that he had experienced a resurgence of his energy and overall health. As he told me, "I'm on a new form of bodybuilding."

Homocysteine and Diet

There's a craze spreading throughout the United States today for high-protein diets, where people eat an enormous amount of animal protein but eat very few plants. I've done a considerable amount of research on the effects of high-protein diets, which I discuss in chapter 11. Those studies reveal what high protein does to the heart. But even before I did my research, scientists knew many of the biochemical effects of high protein on the body, and very few of them, if any, were good.

One of the things scientists have known for some time is that high protein consumption elevates homocysteine, an amino acid that causes changes in the arteries and the blood that significantly increase a person's chances of suffering a heart attack or stroke. There is an ongoing study at Harvard University called the Nurses' Health Study, where researchers have been following the health of approximately 80,000 women for more than 10 years, since 1989. Scientists have found that women with high homocysteine levels have three times the rate of heart disease than women with low homocysteine (Willett 2001). Here are some of the reasons why.

Elevated Homocysteine Injures Your Arteries

When homocysteine enters the blood, it combines with LDL cholesterol to form LDL-complex (LDLc-homocysteine thiolactone), an extremely irritating compound that gets inside your arteries and deforms the artery tissue. It's very common for people with high homocysteine as well to have high LDL levels.

Once the LDL-complex enters the artery wall, the immune system sends monocytes and macrophages to gobble up, or phagocytize, the homocysteine and LDL. That does two things: it turns the immune cells into foam cells, which either create new plaques or make existing plaques bigger; and it triggers an even greater inflammatory reaction inside your arteries. More immune cells arrive on the scene, and a battle rages inside the artery tissue. Soon, the artery tissue swells with immune cells, chemical messengers, and oxidants.

More Homocysteine, More Oxidants

Oxidants, also called free radicals, are highly reactive oxygen molecules that cause molecules, cells, and tissues to become deformed. Immune cells release oxidants to destroy disease-causing agents, such as bacteria and viruses. Most of us have some bacteria circulating in our bloodstreams and hiding away in various places in the body, among them bacteria that cause gingivitis, candidiasis, pneumonia, and various strains of bacteria in the gut. The immune system recognizes them and attacks them with, among other things, oxidants.

High-fat diets are one cause of the production of oxidants, as are elevated levels of homocysteine. The combination of immune cells, high-fat foods, and elevated homocysteine levels causes the blood and artery tissues to be flooded with oxidants. These oxidants cause the decay of LDL particles inside the artery wall. The decaying LDL sets off an even greater immune reaction inside the artery, which leads to more inflammation, more oxidation, and bigger and bigger plaques.

Meanwhile, even as it stimulates plaques to grow, homocysteine also has a vasoconstrictive effect on arteries, meaning it causes them to narrow. Essentially, an artery should expand and contract as needed to regulate the amount of blood that flows through it. Several chemical changes in the blood cause the artery either to expand or contract. As homocysteine levels get higher, they trigger a chemical reaction that forces arteries to narrow. But in an artery in which plaques are growing, any narrowing can be dangerous. A large plaque combined with a narrowing artery increases the likelihood that blood flow will be blocked, which could bring on a heart attack or stroke.

And More Clots, Too

Actually, things can even get worse, impossible as that may seem. Elevated homocysteine increases the blood's viscosity and its tendency to form clots. As you will recall, clots, or thrombi, are the primary cause behind most heart attacks and strokes. When a plaque erupts, a thrombus forms over the open wound in the artery, just as a scab forms over an open cut. If that thrombus is large enough, it can block blood flow to the heart. If the clot breaks free from the plaque (technically it is an embolus if it detaches), it can move through the artery until it gets lodged in a narrow passageway and blocks blood flow. Either way, you've got a serious condition—very likely, a coronary event. Anything that increases the blood's viscosity and tendency to form bigger clots is therefore a dangerous factor in the chain of events that leads to a heart attack or stroke.

Essentially, homocysteine exacerbates conditions at both ends of the problem: it promotes the formation of plaques to begin with, and then it makes the clots bigger when the plaques explode. Homocysteine is now considered to be one of the major risk factors in heart disease. In fact, there are some researchers today who consider homocysteine levels to be at least as important as blood cholesterol levels.

High Meat, High Protein: High Homocysteine

All of which means that you definitely do not want to have elevated homocysteine levels in your blood. But that's exactly what happens when you eat too much protein. Protein drives up homocysteine levels. Here's how.

The protein from meat, eggs, cheese, and other dairy products increases an amino acid called methionine, which is converted to homocysteine. The higher the methionine, the higher the homocysteine. The body uses folic acid and vitamins B_6 and B_{12} to break down homocysteine and convert it into harmless amino acids. Essentially, these vitamins keep homocysteine in check. However, when homocysteine is high, the body requires greater quantities of folic acid and vitamins B_6 and B_{12}. When the body's stores of those vitamins diminish, homocysteine levels rise.

Folic acid and vitamin B_6 are found primarily in plant foods, most notably in green vegetables and whole grains. Without those foods in your diet, the odds are great that you won't get enough folic acid and vitamin B_6 to keep homocysteine levels low. Vitamin B_{12} is derived from bacteria and tends to be concentrated in animal foods. Since people with high homocysteine levels are essentially being poisoned by animal foods, I prefer that vitamin B_{12} be derived from a supplement, at least while you are on the Phase 1 diet. But since Phase 2 allows animal foods to be consumed daily, a B_{12} supplement will no longer be necessary.

On high-protein diets, people eat large quantities of protein but only small amounts of plant foods, so methionine and homocysteine levels are high and folic acid and vitamin B_6 levels are low. That is a heart disease–producing combination.

On the other hand, diets rich in plant foods and low in animal foods are rich in vitamin B_6 and folic acid and low in methionine, so they do not produce high levels of homocysteine. In fact, such diets are also low in saturated fat, calories, and triglycerides—all risk factors for heart disease.

The researchers at the Harvard Nurses' Study have shown that women who consumed the highest amounts of folic acid and vitamin B_6 had only half the risk of dying of a heart attack as women with the lowest intakes of these vitamins.

In Phase 1, I recommend avoiding animal food entirely, instead taking a one-a-day supplement that includes folic acid and vitamins B_6 and B_{12}. The diet that I recommend is rich in folic acid and vitamin B_6. When coupled with the supplement, it also provides those vitamins in abundance, along with optimal levels of vitamin B_{12}. On the Phase 2 diet, I permit limited amounts of animal foods, which means you will get plenty of vitamin B_{12} from the diet alone. You'll also get an abundance of vitamin B_6 and folic acid. In Phase 2, the supplement is optional, but I still believe it's a good thing, especially if you have been on a diet in the past that included high quantities of animal foods.

Have Your Homocysteine Checked

As you might expect, I recommend that everyone have their homocysteine levels checked when they have a physical. Normal homocysteine ranges from 4 to 12 micromoles per liter of blood, or µmol/L. I test all my patients for homocysteine and I like to see their homocysteine levels come down to 10 µmol/L or lower.

According to some studies, every 5 µmol/L increase in homocysteine represents a 60 to 80 percent increase in the risk of heart disease. That puts you in the high-risk category for a heart attack or stroke.

Other research has shown that a 5 µmol/L increase in homocysteine is the equivalent of a 20 mg/dL increase in blood cholesterol. That's a lot, especially when you consider that the National Heart, Lung, and Blood Institute has shown that a 1 percent increase in cholesterol amounts to a

2 percent increase in your risk of heart disease. If your blood cholesterol level is 200 mg/dL and you increase it by 20 mg/dL, you've essentially increased your cholesterol level by 10 percent and your risk of heart disease by 20 percent! No matter how you cut it, elevated homocysteine levels are extremely dangerous.

Antioxidants: Keeping You Young and Healthy (Not to Mention, Alive)

The way to control homocysteine is to reduce protein consumption and increase your consumption of vegetables, beans, fruit, and whole grains. By eating more plant foods, you will improve your body's biochemistry in a multitude of ways—not least by getting lots of folic acid, vitamin B_6, and antioxidants. The first two will reduce homocysteine levels; the third will inhibit its negative effects.

Homocysteine does much of its damage by being a big source of oxidants, which are the driving force behind most major illnesses, including heart disease, cancer, Alzheimer's disease, Parkinson's disease, cataracts, arthritis, asthma, and most other degenerative diseases. They are also the reason our skin wrinkles and our muscles and organs wither.

Perhaps you remember the Stephen King best-seller *Thinner* (it also became a popular film) about a man who made people instantly become old and withered simply by touching them. That, basically, is what oxidants do to your cells and the LDL particles in your blood.

Oxidants cause substances in your body to rapidly age and wither. They force otherwise benign LDL particles to break down and become rancid. At that point, your immune system reacts and triggers an inflammatory reaction inside your blood vessels. Oxidants can turn healthy cells into nonfunctioning scar tissue. If they interact with or touch a cell's DNA, they can turn a normal, healthy cell into a mutation, which in some cases can become cancerous.

How Oxidants Kill

How do oxidants make cholesterol and tissues wither? Essentially, by causing molecules to lose electrons. In order to maintain stability, the atoms within a molecule must have the same number of electrons revolving outside their nuclei as they have protons inside. When the atoms in a molecule lose electrons, the molecule becomes unstable and starts to break down. In an attempt to stop this process of decay, a molecule often tries to steal electrons from a neighboring molecule. If successful, the neighbor becomes unstable, which in turn causes that unstable molecule to steal electrons from its neighbor. The series of thefts creates a kind of biochemical chaos within the decaying cells. Some of these cells become nonfunctional scar tissue. Others die, and still others can become malignant. Cancer feeds on oxidants; it needs them to survive. So after a cancer cell manifests or a tumor appears, the disease requires a steady flow of oxidants to stay alive and grow.

Because oxidants arise from immune activity and normal metabolism—simply breathing in oxygen and utilizing it as fuel causes some oxidation—we cannot escape all of their effects. Fortunately, however, the body has many protective mechanisms to guard against the damage oxidants do to cells, DNA, and organs. What we must limit is our exposure to environmental oxidants. The big sources in our everyday lives are dietary fat, cigarette smoke, ultraviolet light from the sun, homocysteine, and chemical pollutants in our air, water, and soil. To a great extent, these are all controllable sources of oxidation: we can limit how much fat we consume; how much cigarette smoke we inhale; how many industrial pollutants, including pesticides, and ultraviolet rays we are exposed to. Another way to guard against the damage done by oxidants is to consume as many antioxidants as we can.

How Antioxidants Protect You from Heart Disease

Antioxidants protect us by donating electrons to unstable molecules, thus restoring stability to LDL, cell membranes, and the DNA of cells. Antioxidants are the big givers, you might say, preventing oxidation and bringing stability and health to tissues and organs.

The antioxidants that have been most closely examined by scientists are the ones most widely known by all of us: vitamins C, E, and beta-carotene, the vegetable precursor of vitamin A. And indeed, studies have shown that people who eat foods rich in these substances show consistently lower rates of disease, especially heart disease, than those who avoid them.

Foods rich in vitamins C and E have consistently been shown to prevent LDL from oxidizing and thus to slow or prevent the formation of atherosclerotic plaques. Other widely known antioxidants include vitamin B_6 and glutathione; the minerals selenium, zinc, copper, and manganese; and an amino acid called L-cysteine.

One study found that people who ate 180 mg of vitamin C a day—the amount found in two stalks of broccoli—had lower rates of heart disease than the national average. They also experienced a significant drop in blood pressure, which is a major risk factor for heart disease, heart attack, and stroke.

The Harvard Nurses' Health Study found that women who eat foods rich in vitamin E and have higher-than-average levels of this vitamin in their blood have the lowest rates of heart disease. The researchers found that women who took 100 international units of vitamin E a day experienced 40 percent fewer heart attacks than those who avoided vitamin E–rich foods and did not take vitamin E supplements.

The study has shown that other antioxidants such as beta-carotene also play a crucial role in the protection of the heart. In the study, women who ate at least five servings of carrots per week had 68 percent fewer strokes than those who ate carrots only once a month.

One of the ways antioxidants protect you from heart disease is by being highly anti-inflammatory. Though all the common antioxidants may inhibit inflammation, studies have shown that vitamin C is particularly powerful at inhibiting the inflammatory response. Some research suggests that vitamin C's anti-inflammation effects may be effective at reducing symptoms in people with arthritis and asthma.

How do you ensure that you'll get enough foods that are rich in antioxidants to protect your health? The goal that most scientists urge people to reach is five servings per day of vegetables, fruits, and whole grains. However, many health authorities encourage people to eat at least seven to nine servings of plant foods per day. On both the Phase 1 and 2 diets, you exceed nine servings per day, which means you get an abundance of antioxidants.

Plant Foods: The Source of Antioxidants—and Health!

When people ask me why I place so much emphasis on vegetables, I am often reminded of the well-known quote from the bank robber John Dillinger. When a reporter asked Mr. Dillinger why he robbed banks, he said, "Because that's where the money is." When people ask me why I emphasize vegetables, I tell them, "Because that's where the nutrition is." That's especially the case with antioxidants.

The source of all nutrition on the planet is, of course, plants. The only reason beef or pork or chicken contain nutrients is because cows and pigs and chickens eat plants. Animal foods contain concentrated amounts of certain nutrients—iron and calcium, for example. They do not provide the broad spectrum of nutrition that plant foods do.

A good example of this is antioxidants. Animal foods are essentially devoid of antioxidants. Plant foods, on the other hand, are literally exploding with antioxidants. The table on pages 87–88 illustrates this point.

Scientists at the U.S. Department of Agriculture Human Nutrition Research Center on Aging, at Tufts University in Boston, have ranked foods according to their antioxidant content. Here is a short list of the best sources of antioxidants, many of which are also highly anti-inflammatory.

- Blueberries—perhaps the greatest source of antioxidants in the food supply
- Concord grape juice—the highest-antioxidant drink available
- Blackberries
- Strawberries
- Prunes
- Cranberry juice
- Green vegetables such as collard greens, kale, and spinach
- Oranges
- Brussels sprouts
- Grapefruits

One of the reasons I emphasize vegetables and fruits during Phase 1 is because these two categories of foods are bursting with nutrients, especially antioxidants.

The truth is, however, that the best-known antioxidants—vitamin C, vitamin E, and beta-carotene—represent a tiny minority of the antioxidants available in food. In addition to these are the substances known as carotenoids that color plant foods. There are as many as 600 carotenoids, and many of them act as antioxidants. Others serve as immune boosters and still

Good Sources of Antioxidants

Beta-carotene (no established RDA; between 10 and 30 mg per day recommended)

Food	Serving Size	Amount (in mg)	Percentage of RDA
Squash	½ cup	16.1	54
Carrots	½ cup	12.2	41
Kale	½ cup	8.2	27
Mustard greens	½ cup	7.3	24
Spinach	½ cup	4.4	15
Brussels sprouts	½ cup	3.4	11
Sweet potato	1 medium	2.9	10

Vitamin C (RDA: 60 mg)

Food	Serving Size	Amount (in mg)	Percentage of RDA
Papaya	1 medium	188	313
Cantaloupe	½ medium	113	188
Chili pepper	½ cup	109	182
Green bell pepper	1 medium	95	158
Strawberries	1 cup	85	142
Oranges	1 medium	70	117
Kale	½ cup	51	85
Broccoli	½ cup	49	82
Grapefruit	½ medium	41	68
Cauliflower	½ cup	34	57
Potato (baked)	1 medium	26	43
Cabbage	½ cup	17	28

Vitamin E (RDA: 10 mg per day)

Food	Serving Size	Amount	Percentage of RDA
Wheat germ	1 cup	20.5	205
Sunflower seeds	1 ounce	14.8	148

Vitamin E (continued)

Food	Serving Size	Amount	Percentage of RDA
Almonds	1 ounce	7.0	70
Sweet potato	1 medium	5.5	55
Kidney beans	½ cup	4.4	44
Pinto beans	½ cup	4.1	41
Peanuts	1 ounce	3.1	31
Mango	1 medium	2.7	27
Asparagus	½ cup	1.8	18
Wild rice	½ cup	1.8	18
Salmon	3 ounces	1.6–1.8	16–18
Mackerel	3 ounces	1.5	15
Brown rice	½ cup	1.2	12
Cod	3 ounces	0.8	8
Shrimp	3 ounces	0.6–3.5	6–35
Pear	1 medium	.83	8.3
Apple	1 medium	0.4	4
Seven-grain bread	1 slice	0.3	3
Wheat	1 cup	0.3	3

others strengthen our cancer-fighting defenses. The same can be said for many of the tens of thousands of compounds known as phytochemicals. Simply by eating carrots, or squash, or green and leafy vegetables, you consume an abundance of immune system–boosting, heart-disease-and-cancer-fighting antioxidants, carotenoids, and phytochemicals. As with antioxidants, scientists maintain that we can get the minimum level of carotenoids and phytochemicals by eating at least five servings of vegetables, fruit, and grains per day. I recommend that you eat at least nine servings, which is easy on the Fleming Phase 1 and Phase 2 diets.

The following foods, from a list published in *The New York Times* (February 21, 1995), provide the most abundant quantities of carotenoids (given in micrograms), in descending order.

Tomato juice	23,564
Kale, cooked	22,610
Collard greens, cooked	18,445
Spinach, cooked, drained	15,385
Sweet potato, cooked	12,848
Swiss chard, cooked	12,488
Watermelon	12,166
Spinach	12,156
Carrots, cooked	11,696
Pumpkin, canned	10,710

What About Supplements?

We know that those who eat foods rich in antioxidants tend to enjoy better health and have lower rates of disease. The question is, do supplements of antioxidants improve health? So far, the scientific evidence seems to be mixed, especially on the question of whether antioxidant supplements prevent heart attacks or strokes. Although researchers are baffled by the mixed results, they make perfect sense to me. Supplements are not going to overcome the pro-inflammatory effects of an unhealthy diet and lifestyle. If you eat a diet rich in fat, processed foods, and animal protein, you're feeding the fires of inflammation three or four times a day. That's especially the case if you sit around all day and are overweight. A little one-a-day vitamin will not counteract all the damage you're doing. It's like throwing a cup of water on a forest fire. Nothing of any significance can be accomplished.

For those who eat a diet that's rich in anti-inflammatory foods, a multivitamin that contains antioxidants may have a more positive effect, or at least appear to have one.

But why do some studies show that antioxidant supplements have a positive result, while others do not? My answer is this: Within a large population, you will find different ways of eating. Some people eat more vegetables and fruits. Others eat at McDonald's on a regular basis. These diverse ways of eating will have vastly different effects on health. Studies tend to look at large populations of people. Within those large groups, dietary patterns, exercise habits, and ways of dealing with stress vary widely. Researchers attempt to control for some of these variations and even conduct statistical analyses that account for some of them, but such wide variety in lifestyles cannot be fully controlled for and thus can easily skew the results.

Interestingly, the Harvard Nurses' Health Study revealed that women who took an antioxidant supplement had lower rates of disease than those who didn't. This fits my analysis, for the simple reason that women tend to take better care of themselves than men, especially men who are single or divorced. Men who live alone tend to eat more fast food and indulge in more suboptimal health habits than women who live alone. Therefore, studies that examine the health patterns of women are more likely to find a positive effect from the consumption of supplements than similar studies of men. Women are more likely to engage in other behaviors that reduce inflammation, including eating more vegetables and fruits. Studies that include men will find much wider diversity of health habits, and therefore are less likely to show clear benefits from supplements. That's one of the reasons why the research turns up mixed results.

Both the Phase 1 and Phase 2 diets of the Fleming Program are rich in antioxidants and anti-inflammatory foods and contain only negligible amounts of pro-inflammatory foods. Therefore, these diets are going to have a profound effect on your heart and overall health, whether you take a supplement or not.

During Phase 1, I recommend that people take a supplement to support and encourage the healing process. But make no mistake, the healing comes from the food. The supplements provide an extra boost.

I recommend a multivitamin-mineral combination that contains folic acid, vitamins B_6 and B_{12}, and a wide array of antioxidants. I recommend that people on Phase 1 get at least 500 to 1,000 mg a day of vitamin C, 400 to 800 international units (IU) of vitamin E, and 200 mcg of selenium.

Homocysteine, Oxidation, and Cancer

An interesting observation made by researchers is that people who are diagnosed with cancer frequently have a high homocysteine level. This makes sense, because a high homocysteine level suggests chronic inflammation and attendant enormous stress on the immune system. In such cases, the immune system simply cannot cope with all the inflammatory reactions taking place throughout the body and simultaneously battle incipient cancer.

Homocysteine is associated with high oxidative stress as well as high inflammation. A diet that is rich in fat and protein but low in fiber and antioxidants elevates both homocysteine and oxidation. Such a diet can trigger the onset of cancer and support its growth, meaning that the diet that elevates homocysteine also creates the foundation for malignancy. Therefore, it's no wonder that people who are diagnosed with cancer often show high homocysteine levels as well.

The best way to protect yourself against the harmful effects of homocysteine is by eating a diet rich in plant foods comprising a wide variety of vegetables, beans, whole grains, and fruit. All of the harmful effects of homocysteine are mitigated, and in many cases prevented entirely, by eating these foods in abundance. With them, you will get optimal amounts of immune system–boosting and cancer-fighting antioxidants, carotenoids, and phytochemicals. When people make the switch from the standard Western diet to the Fleming Program Phase 1 and 2 diets, they experience a transformation that they would not have believed possible.

It Can All Be Reversed

Gary, a 39-year-old postal worker, came to see me in May 2001. He suffered from arrhythmia (irregular heartbeat), chest pain, and bouts of weakness. Gary was married and had two young children, both in grammar school. He stood just under six feet tall and weighed 195 pounds, so he was not grossly overweight but a bit chubby. In addition to documented heart disease, Gary also had stomach ulcers. After a battery of tests and a SPECT test of his heart, I discovered that Gary had a cholesterol level of 153 mg/dL, which was not bad at all, especially given his high-fat, high-processed-foods diet. He had a triglycerides level of 148, also well within healthy ranges. But the SPECT test showed significant heart disease. His left ventricle, or lower left chamber, was damaged from lack of blood flow, and there was significant obstruction from cholesterol plaque in his left anterior descending coronary artery and right coronary artery. In addition, his homocysteine level was 14.5 µmol/L—way out of the healthy range.

I put him on the Phase 1 diet, and he followed it religiously. He also walked every day. Three times a week, he also carried small, five-pound hand weights to promote upper-body strength. By July he had lost 20 pounds—all of

REVERSING HEART DISEASE ON
THE FLEMING PROGRAM:
STEPS 5 AND 6

Step 5. Achieve optimal homocysteine levels by eliminating animal proteins during Phase 1, limit them during Phase 2, and increase folic acid and vitamins B_6 and B_{12} by eating a plant-based diet and taking a daily vitamin-mineral-antioxidant supplement.

Step 6. Increase antioxidant intake by eating a plant-based diet and taking a daily supplement that includes optimal levels of antioxidants.

*

it "baby fat," as he called it. Not only was he lean, I told him, but you could also clearly see muscle development in his arms and upper body. He had no chest pain, no dysrhythmia, and no discomfort from his stomach ulcers. His cholesterol level fell to 130 mg/dL and his triglyceride level to 125 mg/dL. His homocysteine level was 9.4 μmol/L, well below 10, which is where I like to see it.

And then the Twin Towers of the World Trade Center were attacked on September 11, 2001, and Gary, like so many thousands of other Americans, fell like those great American buildings. Gary stopped following Phase 1 and began eating what he called "comfort foods"—ice cream, pizza, and processed foods, including doughnuts. He also suffered from a great deal of stress for several weeks when the anthrax scare hit post offices around the country. Who could blame him? But his health was clearly deteriorating. His chest pain returned, as did his ulcers. We had a long talk about the stresses he was facing and the effect of those "comfort foods" on his heart. By mid-October, he had returned to the Phase 1 regimen, and within two weeks he had no chest pain, no ulcer discomfort, and no arrhythmia.

By the spring of 2002, Gary's homocysteine levels had fallen to 7.3! All his old symptoms had disappeared. Confirming all the progress he had made, a new SPECT test showed remarkable improvement of blood flow to his heart, and he even regained heart function in the area of his left ventricle. The love of his family and his friends, along with his diet and exercise program, had brought him through one of the most stressful periods of his life. And his health was better than it had been in decades.

Growth Factors, Fibrinogen, and Lipoprotein (a)

IN THE FALL OF 1997, AT THE ANNUAL meeting of the American Heart Association (AHA) in Dallas, Texas, I told a group of fellow physicians that I believed hormone replacement therapy (HRT) increased a woman's chances of having a heart attack. HRT, I said, is probably one of the reasons women have more heart attacks after menopause. I went even further. I expected the data from a forthcoming study examining the effects of HRT on women to prove my hypothesis correct.

This was not the first time I had said such a thing, nor would it be the last. I had presented a paper on the subject at a medical meeting in Istanbul in June 1997, and would do so again in Lisbon in June 1998.

At the AHA meeting, my colleagues' reactions to my statement ranged from outright laughter to silent rebuke. Judging by the looks on some of the faces, I was not someone who should be taken seriously. Everyone knew that HRT was an effective therapy for the prevention of heart disease and osteoporosis, as well as the alleviation of menopausal symptoms. To offer a contrary opinion was to reveal one's ignorance.

The forthcoming study I was referring to was the Hormone Estrogen Replacement Study, or HERS trial, the results of which were to be published just a week after that AHA meeting where I had made my incredible statement. The HERS data was published in the *Journal of the American Medical Association* and, just as I had predicted, the data showed that HRT did indeed increase a woman's risk of heart attack, especially during the early years of treatment. The HERS trial showed that the risk fell off as time went on, but by that time the damage had already been done. A follow-up study, known as HERS II, confirmed the earlier findings and then compounded the heresy by showing that there was no reduction in the risk of heart attack for women who continued taking HRT after the first three years of treatment.

Because the belief in HRT was so deeply embedded, the HERS trial was greeted with widespread skepticism and even disbelief among many medical doctors. "More research is needed," was the loudest response. By the year 2000, hormone replacement therapy was being used by more than 20 million women in the United States alone.

However, the shaky faith in HRT collapsed overnight when the flagship research project (conducted by the National Institutes of Health) known as the Women's Health Initiative (WHI) released its data in the summer of 2002. The Women's Health Initiative was the largest and most rigorously designed study ever done on the effects of hormone replacement therapy on women. What the study found was that HRT increases a woman's risk of heart attack, stroke, and breast and uterine cancers. In fact, the researchers had to stop the study prematurely to protect the health of the participants, because the data were showing a clear relationship between the drugs being studied and the increased rates of heart attacks (Writing Group for the Women's Health Initiative Investigators 2002).

HRT does offer some small protection against bone loss after menopause, but that protection is much smaller than previously thought, and the liabilities far outweigh it. Besides, as researchers across the country have noted, there are other methods for preventing osteoporosis that are more effective and do not pose the same risk for heart disease or cancer. HRT also reduces some of the symptoms associated with menopause, such as hot flashes, night sweats, and mood swings. These are the only claims that manufacturers of HRT drugs can make.

With the release of the WHI data, HRT went from being an almost universally celebrated treatment to one that was dropped as if it had been suddenly revealed as arsenic therapy. How did I know five years ago that HRT was bad for the heart? In fact, the evidence was staring us in the face all the while. The key clue was fibrinogen, which promotes blood clotting and increases inflammation. It was well known that HRT elevated a woman's fibrinogen levels. When I saw that, I knew HRT would have two devastating effects on women's hearts and arteries. Doctors and researchers who supported HRT made the argument that estrogen protected women from heart disease. Estrogens that are produced naturally, by a woman's body, do appear to protect women from heart disease. But we are talking about the effects of HRT, not of the estrogens produced by a woman's ovaries. And as far as I was concerned, the fact that HRT elevates fibrinogen, promotes blood clotting, and triggers inflammation made the results from both the HERS and the WHI trials a foregone conclusion.

Fibrinogen: Balance Is Essential to Heart Health

Fibrinogen is formed in the liver and is one of several clotting proteins that combine with blood platelets to help the blood coagulate to form a scab and halt bleeding from wounds. Under normal conditions, clotting proteins are dormant. However, whenever an injury occurs in your body, including an injury to one or more of your arteries, these proteins spring into action. They quickly go through a series of chemical transformations to form fibrinogen. At the same time, blood platelets arrive on the scene of the injury to help bind the wound. Under healthy conditions, the fibrinogen makes the platelets sticky, causing them to adhere to one another and form a clot that covers the wound and begins the healing process. But when fibrinogen is elevated, too many platelets can bind together, making for a much larger mass inside the artery pathway. That mass, of course, is a clot. If the clot is large enough, it can block the blood vessel entirely, causing a heart attack or stroke.

Several things can happen to cause an injury to your artery wall and trigger the chain of events that lead to clot formation. For most people, that injury occurs when high cholesterol, homocysteine, and immune cells combine to form an inflammatory reaction inside the walls of your arteries. Another common source of injury is high blood pressure, which causes fissures to form inside the artery tissue, which the body recognizes as wounds. Medical procedures such as the implantation of a stent, cardiac catheterization, and balloon angioplasty typically also leave the artery injured and inflamed.

It's crucial for your body to maintain the right fibrinogen level. Too much and you're likely to form clots; too little and you're at risk of suffering a hemorrhage and bleeding to death. The normal fibrinogen range is 200 to 400 mg/dL, but most doctors want to see your fibrinogen levels below 350.

Several factors raise fibrinogen, and, not surprisingly, nearly all of them are associated with higher rates of heart disease. Among them are cigarette smoking, lack of exercise, and high homocysteine levels, which inhibit the breakdown and elimination of fibrinogen from the body. A high-fat diet and infections, including conditions such as gingivitis (gum disease), also increase fibrinogen levels.

Squarely in the midst of all these unhealthful behaviors and conditions is HRT. This should have been a case of guilt by association, meaning that, if HRT were having the same effects as cigarette smoking and lack of exercise, it should have been considered dubious from the start. But we were blinded by the illusory benefits from these drugs. The WHI study removed those blinders from our eyes.

Dr. Bruce Ettinger, a researcher at the Kaiser Permanente medical care program in Oakland, California, told the *New York Times* (September 3, 2002): "WHI changed the way we think about estrogen. This is not a drug to be used for prevention. Giving the drug to a lot of healthy women is not the right thing to do."

Heart Disease: The Number One Killer of Women

Both men and women must be concerned about elevated fibrinogen levels. But women especially must be aware that fibrinogen is an independent—and extremely important—risk factor for heart disease, especially in light of new research on HRT.

Right now, 9 million women suffer from heart disease, and this year 500,000 women will die from the illness. About 250,000 women die annually from heart attacks alone. Compare that to the 40,500 women killed each year from breast cancer and you start to realize just how big a problem heart disease really is and, in comparison, how little attention it gets.

Many women have high cholesterol levels. By the time the average woman reaches the age of 45, her cholesterol level is 220 mg/dL. Obviously, that's well into the danger zone. Yet despite their cholesterol levels, premenopausal women have far lower rates of heart disease than men. The reason, doctors believe, is the presence of estrogen, which tends to increase HDL cholesterol and lower the impact of LDL on a woman's coronary arteries. Unfortunately, the protective effects of estrogen vanish at menopause, when estrogen levels fall substantially. At that point, cholesterol levels in women tend to go up, as does the incidence of heart attacks and strokes. By the time the average woman reaches the age of 65, her chances of dying of a heart attack are slightly greater than the average man's.

In addition to protecting a woman's heart, estrogen is essential for the health and strength of her bones. Estrogen's counterpart in men is testosterone, the male hormone, which men need to maintain bone strength and density. For both sexes, the skeleton tends to grow stronger and thicker up until the age of about 35, at which point people start losing bone mass at a rate of about 1 percent per year. After menopause, when estrogen levels fall, the danger of osteoporosis increases as bone loss speeds up to about 5 percent a year. That can be a substantial and dangerous condition, especially if a woman is small-boned already.

Since estrogen seems to be essential to both heart and skeletal health, doctors argued that replacing it after menopause would protect a woman's heart and her bones. There were also other reasons to use HRT to replace hormones. Menopause brings with it a host of distressing symptoms, including night sweats, hot flashes, loss of tissue elasticity, vaginal dryness, and vaginal atrophy. HRT seemed like an answer to all of these problems.

Hormone replacement therapy has been used for 60 years; the Food and Drug Administration approved its use in 1942. Initially, estrogen alone was replaced, but estrogen replacement resulted in a dramatic increase risk of uterine and endometrial cancers. Researchers found that women who took estrogens alone had up to 14 times greater risk of contracting uterine cancer than those who did not take estrogen. Women who took estrogens also experienced increased risk of contracting diabetes and gallbladder disease.

In order to protect women against the cancerous effects of estrogen replacement, progesterone was added to the HRT formula. Unfortunately, progesterone increases fibrinogen, promotes increased blood clotting, and lowers HDL. Because HRT and birth control pills—also a source of estrogen and progesterone—raised fibrinogen levels, doctors routinely warned women who received HRT or took birth control pills not to smoke. Cigarette smoking not only raises fibrinogen but also causes arteries to constrict, a very dangerous combination. When you add HRT to that mix, you get a formula for heart attacks and strokes.

In addition, studies also revealed that the estrogen-progesterone formula increased a woman's risk of developing breast cancer. All of these effects seemed to reduce HRT's heart-protecting benefits, but doctors nonetheless kept prescribing the hormones in order to prevent heart disease. That is, until the WHI study cleared away the misconceptions.

In the wake of the HERS and WHI studies, the American Heart Association warned women not to take hormone therapy as a way of preventing heart attack and stroke. Hormone replacement therapy, the AHA said, may do women more harm than good.

The June 13, 2001, issue of the *Journal of the American Medical Association* (JAMA) reported that studies showing HRT's protective benefits had very likely been misinterpreted. Women who took HRT probably took much better care of themselves generally than those who did not take the drugs. These women were more likely to avoid smoking, engage in daily exercise, and eat a more plant-centered diet, all of which reduce a woman's risk of osteoporosis. The benefits previously associated with HRT, scientists now believe, very likely were caused by these healthy lifestyles and not by the hormone therapy.

Liver Health and the Heart

An old ditty about the interconnectedness of the human body goes something like this: "The knee bone's connected to the shin bone, the shin bone's connected to the ankle bone, the ankle bone's connected to the foot bone . . . ," and so on. Well, in the case of heart disease, we could sing a similar song, one that goes: "The liver's connected to the arteries, and the arteries are connected to the heart organ . . ." In other words, the health of your arteries and heart depends on the health of your liver. Unfortunately, the standard Western diet generates enormous inflammation within the liver, which damages the organ and causes it to produce abnormal amounts of chemicals that gradually destroy the arteries and the heart. In all too many cases, heart disease begins in the liver. Here's what happens.

The chemicals fibrinogen, homocysteine, and C-reactive protein—all of which directly affect the health of your arteries and heart—are produced by the liver when it becomes inflamed and imbalanced, usually due to high quantities of pro-inflammatory foods. Recently, scientists have discovered that yet another chemical produced by the liver also plays a vital role in the etiology of heart disease. That chemical is lipoprotein (a), often referred to as "lipoprotein little a" and written "Lp(a)."

Lp(a) promotes clot formation by preventing the breakdown of fibrinogen, thereby increasing fibrinogen levels and making the blood more viscous and more likely to form clots. Lp(a) is very much like LDL cholesterol, meaning it plays a role in the creation of inflammation within the artery. It also has a rather unique characteristic which makes it even more treacherous: a kind of Velcro-like surface that makes it adhere to plaques and to other plaque-promoting substances, such as LDL cholesterol. The sticky Lp(a) acts like a sticky fly strip hanging from a ceiling. Once it attaches itself to a plaque, it snags all kinds of plaque-promoting substances, making the plaque bigger and more likely to block blood flow to the heart or brain.

Individually, fibrinogen and Lp(a) are now considered independent risk factors for heart disease. Recent studies suggest that high levels of Lp(a) may be especially dangerous in causing heart attacks that occur in the morning. Most heart attacks take place between the hours of 6 A.M. and noon, but many people also suffer heart attacks later in the day or evening hours. Japanese researchers compared two groups of people who had suffered heart attacks at different times of the day, one group, in the morning, and the other, after the noon hour. The researchers found that those who suffered morning heart attacks had higher levels of Lp(a) in their bloodstreams than those who had them later in the day.

Other studies have shown that Lp(a) may be one of the most predictive factors when determining a person's risk of heart attack, stroke, and immediate closure of the artery after medical procedures, such as the insertion of a stent or balloon angiopasty.

Like fibrinogen and other clotting proteins, Lp(a) arises in the blood when there is injury to the artery. Lp(a) and other clotting proteins attempt to heal the artery wall by forming a plaque as a protective shield over a wound in the vessel. The more injuries there are to arteries, the more fibrinogen and Lp(a) are present, and the more atherosclerosis.

Interestingly, Lp(a) and fibrinogen have exactly the opposite effect on the arteries as the antioxidants, especially vitamin C. Lp(a) attempts to cover the wound with a volatile scab that is prone to rupture. Antioxidants reduce or eliminate inflammation from the artery wall. They restore the artery's integrity, flexibility, and strength. Antioxidants, when consumed as part of a low-fat, high-fiber diet, restore the smooth, healthy surface of the artery.

The healthy range for Lp(a) is less than 30 mg/dL of blood; anything above 30 should prompt you and your doctor to make changes in your regimen. The first thing you should do if your Lp(a) is high is go on the Phase 1 diet of the Fleming Program. The combination of low-fat, low-inflammatory foods and the abundance of antioxidants, carotenoids, and phytochemicals will immediately lower your LDL cholesterol, homocysteine, and C-reactive protein levels. It will also start the healing process in your liver.

I have found that it takes about three months to bring Lp(a) down into the healthy range. The reason, I theorize, is because it takes that long for the inflammation in the liver to be significantly reduced and for the organ to regain its biochemical balance. You may be heartened to know that even when more than half of the liver's functional capacity has been lost, virtually all of it can be regained through proper diet and lifestyle. The liver is essential for life, and nature has equipped it with marvelous regenerative powers. The Fleming Program can do a great deal to bring the liver back to health.

Lowering Fibrinogen and Other Inflammatory Markers

One of the best ways to lower your fibrinogen levels is to exercise. Moderate exercise has been shown repeatedly to lower fibrinogen, as well as C-reactive protein and Lp(a). A study published in the *Archives of Internal Medicine* (Abramson 2002) examined 3,638 healthy men and women 40 years of age and older. They were tested for their C-reactive protein, fibrinogen, and white blood cell count, which is usually high in people with higher levels of inflammation. Those who exercised 22 times per month or more had significantly lower levels of inflammatory markers than those who exercised zero to three times per month. Another study, published in the *American Journal of Public Health* similarly showed a reduction in lipoprotein (a) and overall incidence of heart disease in people who exercised regularly (Martin 1999). The exercise program described in chapter 4 can lower your inflammation by lowering fibrinogen, C-reactive protein, and Lp(a) levels.

In addition to exercise, certain spices can be helpful in lowering your inflammatory markers, especially fibrinogen. Tumeric and its relative, ginger root, both lower leukotriene levels and reduce inflammation. Turmeric (*Curcuma longa*) is a common spice that is traditional in Indian curry dishes but can be used widely in many kinds of soups, stews, and as a condiment in bean and grain dishes. It has been used safely in cooking for thousands of years and has been shown to be a potent antioxidant. The Spanish researchers A. Ramirez-Bosca and A. Soler also found that turmeric dramatically lowers fibrinogen levels without any negative side effects. Ramirez-Bosca and Soler studied the effects of a tumeric extract, curcumin, on eight subjects with fibrinogen levels as high as 800 mg/dL. After 15 days of treatment, fibrinogen levels were halved (Ramirez-Bosca 2000).

Researchers in Israel have found that people who regularly eat turmeric have lower risks of urinary-tract cancers, including those of the bladder and prostate.

Growth Factors

Growth factors are a class of chemicals that occur naturally in the body. Their task, as their name suggests, is to stimulate growth, meaning they promote cell proliferation and tissue development. A certain amount of cell growth is essential for all of us, especially infants, children, and pregnant women. The key is balance, of course.

Dangers of Growth Factors

Problems arise when growth factors stimulate excessive growth, so that they stimulate cells to multiply even when the cells are not needed. That's when growth factors give rise to immune and inflammatory reactions, which can lead to several kinds of illnesses, including heart disease, rheumatoid arthritis, and cancer. In the case of heart disease, growth factors cause inflammation and swelling of the coronary arteries, eventually leading to plaques and unstable clots. In the case of cancer, growth factors have an effect similar to that of gasoline thrown on a fire. They fuel the life and strength of cancer cells and tumors. Of the growth factors that exist in the human body, the most potentially dangerous is insulin-like growth factor 1, known as IGF-1. This chemical plays a role in heart disease, bowel disorders, arthritis, and cancers of the breast and prostate. In addition to triggering inflammatory reactions and cell growth, elevated IGF-1 also causes constriction of blood vessels, which narrows arteries.

Essentially, there are two causes of elevated growth-factor levels: chronically high insulin levels, caused by consuming too many calories and consuming cow's milk and cow's milk products. Though researchers are still exploring the question, growth factors may also be promoted by high-protein diets. More work needs to be done before that question is settled, however.

DANGER NUMBER ONE: TOO MANY CALORIES

What we do know for sure is that insulin levels become elevated when we eat too many calories. Of course, it's almost impossible not to eat too many calories when you eat processed foods and refined sugar, both of which cause insulin to spike. A fraction of that excess insulin is then converted to IGF-1. The more calories you eat, the higher your insulin levels and the more IGF-1 you have, making you likely to suffer all the myriad consequences of high IGF-1, which include high risk of heart disease and cancer. Type 2 diabetics—who usually are overweight, consume excess calories, have high insulin levels, and are insulin-resistant—usually turn out to have high growth-factor levels, including IGF-1.

Since most Americans eat an abundance of processed foods, and many Americans are overweight, it's fair to assume that most Americans have chronically elevated growth factors. This explains, at least in part, why we have such high levels of heart disease, cancer, arthritis, and other inflammation-caused illnesses.

Interestingly, inflammation itself gives rise to growth factors. Here again, we have a viscious cycle in which certain elements of the diet increase growth factors, inflammation, and rates of illness. Once that inflammation manifests, it triggers the production of more growth factors, which fuels the inflammatory cycle. This is one of the ways coronary heart disease feeds itself—by promoting growth factors on its own.

DANGER NUMBER TWO: THE SACRED COW

The other way to elevate growth factors is to consume dairy products. Studies have consistently shown that consumption of cow's milk is linked to cancer, including cancers of the prostate and breast. Presumably, that link between milk and cancer could be IGF-1. Cow's milk, cheese, yogurt, and butter naturally contain IGF-1. However, research has shown that cows treated with genetically engineered recombinant bovine growth hormone (rBGH) have significantly higher quantities of IGF-1 than untreated cows. Bovine growth hormone is used to stimulate greater milk production. After injection, the animals produce about 10 percent more milk than untreated cows.

Monsanto, the manufacturer of rBGH, says that about a third of the dairy cows in the United States have been treated with rBGH, but farmers across the country have resisted the drug, and activists say that only between 5 and 7 percent of the dairy cows have been injected with the hormone. Unfortunately, however, milk from untreated cows is mixed in large transportation tanks with the milk from treated cows, which means that a much greater percentage of today's milk supply has been tainted with this drug. Nevertheless, when you eat dairy products, you still get higher levels of IGF-1. You just get more from the rBGH-treated animals.

Bovine growth hormone is not the only reason to avoid milk products, nor is it the only reason that cow's milk causes inflammation. Most of the dairy herd has been treated with antibiotics (to prevent disease) and steroids (to make the animals bigger and more productive). Not surprisingly, milk products routinely turn up trace residues of both antibiotics and steroids.

The Food and Drug Administration has maintained that the milk from rBGH-treated animals is identical to that of animals that are untreated. Most states do not require treated milk to be labeled as such, which has infuriated and galvanized farmers across the country. Individual states have created their own laws that allow farmers to advertise their milk as untreated. Milk products labeled "organic" are from cows that have not been treated with rBGH or injected with antibiotics or steroids.

Another problem is that whole milk is high in fat, including saturated fat, which promotes heart disease and is linked to cancer, diabetes, and other serious illnesses.

Furthermore, in 1992 the *New England Journal of Medicine* reported that bovine albumin peptide, one of the proteins in cow's milk, can trigger an autoimmune response in sensitive children and can cause type 1 (juvenile onset) diabetes. This and other studies have shown that milk proteins attach themselves to the pancreas, the organ that produces insulin. Recognizing the milk proteins as a threat to health, the immune system attacks these bovine peptides, but in the process also destroys the insulin-producing cells of the pancreas, thus rendering the organ incapable of making insulin. The result is incurable diabetes. When scientists examine populations of people around the world, they discover a strong association between milk consumption and diabetes.

An unknown percentage of the population clearly has an adverse reaction to milk products. Among those people are many children who suffer autoimmune and inflammatory reactions after consuming dairy foods. Those reactions frequently occur in the intestinal tract and can give rise to an array of conditions, including iron-deficiency anemia, leaky gut syndrome, allergies, asthma, and various types of digestive disorders.

Much of the world's population is lactose intolerant, meaning they are unable to digest lactose, the sugar in milk products. Populations that are lactose intolerant include a high percentage of Asians, Africans, Latin Americans, Native Americans, and about 15 percent of Caucasians. These people lack the enzyme lactase, which is needed to break down and digest lactose. After consuming dairy products, lactose-intolerant people can suffer from gastrointestinal disorders including diarrhea, indigestion, heartburn, and flatulence.

Whenever the health effects of dairy products for Americans are questioned, the immediate worry is calcium sources and osteoporosis. Suffice it to say for now that dairy products are not an ideal source of calcium, largely because the protein in dairy foods causes calcium to be lost from the body. It's also important to keep in mind that epidemiological research has shown that the populations throughout the world with the highest rates of osteoporosis also consume the highest amounts of dairy foods. Populations that do not consume dairy foods but instead get their calcium largely from plant sources tend to have extremely low rates of osteoporosis.

How to Reduce Growth-Factor Levels

The best way to bring your growth-factor levels back into a healthy range is to eat a diet that does the following:

- Keeps calorie consumption down.
- Keeps insulin levels low.
- Fills you up and creates satiety and satisfaction.

The Fleming Program Phase 1 and 2 diets do all three. This program is loaded with flavor, fiber, water, and nutrition, all of which combine to create fullness and deep satisfaction. The fiber and water have no calories, but together they provide lots of bulk. They fill your stomach, but without adding calories. That means that you're going to lose weight. Low calorie consumption and weight loss will bring down your growth-factor levels, including that of IGF-1. Because the foods are also rich in nutrients and the recipes delicious, the program also provides maximum flavor and satisfaction. Give yourself a chance to regain your health by following the program. Witness for yourself the transformation that is possible, as the following Fleming patient experienced.

Gene's Story

Gene, a 68-year-old retired autoworker, arrived in my office in the spring of 2002 suffering from severe chest pain, which came on him four times a day. His cholesterol level was 225 mg/dL, his triglycerides were at 240 mg/dL, and his C-reactive protein level was 0.8 (normal is below 0.5). His fibrinogen was 477 mg/dL (normal is 200 to 400), his blood sugar was 121 mg/dL (normal is 70 to 105). He was nearly 20 pounds overweight and had high blood pressure. To top it all off, Gene had claudication, meaning insufficient circulation in his legs. He experienced painful cramping in his legs, and his feet and toes were constantly cold. If the condition did not improve, he stood a very real chance of losing some portion of one or both legs.

Gene had already suffered two heart attacks and had had triple-vessel coronary bypass surgery in 1993. When he came to see me, only one artery was substantially open; the other two were about 80 percent closed. Needless to say, Gene was extremely ill. He had been on a multitude of medications, he had had surgery, and he had essentially run out of medical options.

Gene had come to me at his wife's insistence. Joan was in fairly good health. Her weight was fine and she had lots of energy—she had been taking good care of herself for most of her life. Gene, on the other hand, was on death's door and he knew it.

Gene's severe suffering proved to be more than enough incentive for him to change his ways of eating and living. After my meeting with Gene and Joan, they went home and literally threw out all the inflammation-producing foods in their refrigerator and pantry. Then they both started the Phase 1 diet, eating only cooked vegetables, salads, and fruit every day. They took a couple of short walks daily and increased their distances slowly and incrementally. By June, Gene had lost 15 pounds and had no more chest pains. By August, his cholesterol level was down to 140 mg/dL; his triglycerides were at 150 mg/dL, and his fibrinogen, C-reactive protein, blood pressure, and blood sugar were all normal. His claudication had cleared up substantially so that he could walk without pain.

REVERSING HEART DISEASE ON THE FLEMING PROGRAM: STEPS 7 AND 8 BRING CLOTTING AND GROWTH FACTORS INTO HEALTHY RANGES WITH PHASE 1 OF THE FLEMING PROGRAM:

Step 7: Fibrinogen levels should be below 300 mg/dL, and lp(a) should fall below 30 mg/dL.

Step 8: IGF-1 should fall below the upper limit (nanograms per milliliter, ng/ml) determined by age and sex (ages 9–15) as shown below.

Age	Male	Female
2 months to 5 years	17–248	17–248
6–8 years	88–474	88–474
9–11 years	110–565	117–771
12–15 years	202–957	261–1096
16–24 years	182–780	182–780
25–39 years	114–492	114–492
40–54 years	90–360	90–360
55 years and older	71–290	71–290

*

Leukotrienes, Complement, and Bacteria

✳

In August 2002, Mary, a native of England who had recently immigrated to the United States, came to see me with a variety of symptoms, the most acute being chest pains. Mary was five feet one inch tall and weighed approximately 120 pounds, so weight was not an issue. Just about everything else was, however. I did a series of tests, including an echocardiogram, a test that uses sound waves to view and diagnose the heart, and a SPECT test of her heart. Both tests revealed that she had significant atherosclerosis in her coronary arteries. She had not had a heart attack, and none of the tissue of the heart was dead, but one area of the heart was so weakened by lack of blood that it was not beating with the same power and function that the rest of the heart possessed.

In addition to her heart disease, Mary had a hypoactive thyroid, meaning her thyroid was producing too little thyroid hormone, the hormone that regulates metabolism. The consequence for Mary was that she suffered from chronic fatigue, dry skin, constipation, and sensitivity to cold, all common side effects of hypothyroidism. Whenever the thyroid is underactive, the pituitary gland boosts production of thyroid-stimulating hormone (TSH), a chemical that acts like a whip on the hindquarters of the thyroid, so to speak. Thus high TSH is a sign of an underactive thyroid.

On top of all of these problems, further tests revealed that Mary had extensive cholesterol plaques in her carotid artery (located in the neck), as well as elevated glucose (blood sugar), cholesterol, triglycerides, homocysteine, Lp(a), C-reactive protein, and leukotrienes.

Leukotrienes, also referred to as interleukins, are chemical messengers produced by immune cells. These messengers relay commands to immune cells to perform tasks, such as to divide and multiply in the face of a threat or to call out lymphocytes or B cells to produce antibodies to fight infections. The problem with leukotrienes is that, when their levels become elevated, they cause a variety of harmful changes within the artery tissue that lead to increased atherosclerosis. Inevitably, high leukotrienes indicate that an acute immune reaction is occurring and that lots of inflammation is being produced.

"Mary, here's the problem," I said. "If I increase the dosages of your medications, or give you new meds, the drugs may mask your symptoms temporarily, but they will not change your fundamental health for the better. In fact, you may even get worse, even as you take the drugs, because you will not have changed the reason you are ill in the first place. What you have to do is radically change your diet and start exercising four or five times a week. Can you do that?" I asked.

"How radical is radical?" she asked me.

"I want you to eat only vegetables and fruit for a few months," I said. "This diet will cause all of the numbers from glucose to leukotrienes to fall. Once that happens, you'll feel great. Your pain will probably disappear, you'll have lots of energy and clarity of mind, and you'll very likely experience a positive emotional state. Can you make that kind of radical dietary change?"

"Only vegetables and fruit?" she asked me. "Why? Am I that sick?"

"Yes, you are," I said. "Your high cholesterol and angina mean that your heart is not getting enough oxygen. At the same time, you've got a lot of inflammation going on in your arteries. That means the plaques in your arteries are probably unstable. One of those plaques could erupt when you least expect it. It could form a clot and you could have a fatal heart attack."

"How long do I have to eat just vegetables and fruit?" Mary asked me.

"Just for a few months," I responded, "until your numbers come down into the normal ranges. Then I'll put you on my Phase 2 program and you'll have much more flexibility with your diet."

"I suppose eating vegetables and fruit for a few months is a lot better than dying," Mary said. "Yes, I can radically change my diet."

Mary was as good as her word. But neither one of us expected the kind of results she experienced nor the speed with which she recovered. After two weeks of Phase 1, all of Mary's numbers declined dramatically. Her test results were as follows:

- Total cholesterol fell from 204 to 181 mg/dL.
- Glucose tolerance (the test for diabetes) dropped from 127 mg/dL to 108 (normal is 70 to 105 mg/dL).
- Triglycerides dropped from 169 to 107 mg/dL (normal is less than 150 mg/dL).
- Thyroid-stimulating hormone (TSH) fell from 9.17 micro international units per milliliter of blood (μIU/mL) to a normal level of 5.22 (normal is 0.35 to 6.90 μIU/mL).
- Homocysteine dropped from 9.7 to 7.9 μmol/L (normal is between 4 and 10 in women and between 4 and 12 in men).
- Lp(a) dropped from 50 to 35 mg/dL (normal is less than 30 mg/dL). This wasn't quite normal as yet, but on the way.
- C-RP fell from 0.6 to 0.3 mg/dL (normal is less than 0.5 mg/dL).
- And perhaps most impressive, the leukotriene levels, especially interleukin-6, a very inflammatory leukotriene, dropped from 21.9 to below 5 picograms/milliliter (normal range is below 9.8 pg/mL).

Meanwhile, because her coronary arteries were opening and allowing more blood to flow, her angina pain disappeared. This was confirmed by an electrocardiogram and a SPECT test, both of which showed improved blood flow to her heart. Even more impressive was that heart tissue that had ceased to function had been recovered and was now showing movement. And all of this occurred between August 16 and August 29! Within three months of adopting Phase 1, all of Mary's numbers had fallen into the ideal ranges and she was off all medication.

The speed of Mary's progress at the outset of her treatment surprised me, but the overall treatment outcome did not, because I have seen it so many times before. Among the many miracles of the human body are its resilience and regenerative capabilities. Given the right circumstances, the human body can heal itself of just about anything. By the "right circumstances," I mean a healing diet, a gentle exercise regimen, a balanced lifestyle, and medical treatment when necessary.

What most of us are coping with today is exactly the opposite set of conditions: a destructive diet, the absence of exercise, and a lifestyle that is extremely stressful. Of those three factors, diet and exercise have the most powerful impact on health. This is especially the case with diet, which drives all the major risk factors, including blood cholesterol, triglycerides, homocysteine, antioxidant levels, fibrinogen, Lp(a), growth factors, and leukotrienes, as you will see in this chapter.

Controlling stress, the third negative condition, is also important, make no mistake. What many people don't realize is that appropriate diet and exercise determine to a great extent how well we deal with stress. Exercise is among the most powerful treatments for relieving stress. A simple walk in the mornings, during the day, and in the evenings can dramatically lower stress levels and clear our minds so that we can be more creative and effective at dealing with the issues we face. Reducing or eliminating beverages that contain caffeine or alcohol, as well as lowering fat intake and eliminating processed foods, especially those that contain sugar, profoundly improves the clarity of the mind and the energy levels of the body. People who believe that stress alone is the problem are generally fooling themselves in order to avoid changing their eating and exercise habits.

Leukotrienes: Essential, But Easily Out of Control

One risk factor that very clearly reveals this connection is the leukotriene level. Leukotrienes, an essential part of the immune system's communication network, rise and fall depending on our dietary choices and the overall health of our arteries. When leukotriene levels are up, you can be sure that the person not only is on a poor diet but also is at high risk of having a heart attack or stroke.

The immune system, composed of approximately 3 trillion cells, is highly organized, extremely powerful, and extremely efficient. One of the ways the immune system maintains its order, power, and efficiency is its ability to communicate across relatively vast distances. To a microscopic cell, the distance between your head and your big toe would seem like hundreds, perhaps thousands, of miles when placed on a human scale. The immune system communicates over these huge distances with an efficiency that should impress any telephone company. This communication is made possible by chemical messengers that are secreted by immune cells, referred to collectively as cytokines.

Leukotrienes, or interleukins, are a subclass of cytokines produced by white blood cells. Leukotrienes are essential to the proper functioning of your body's defenses. In a healthy person, the activity of leukotrienes is usually a very good thing, especially when that person encounters a pathogen of some type. Remember the last time you had the flu or a common cold and wanted to get rid of it as quickly as you could? Your leukotrienes were giving orders to your immune cells to become more numerous, more aggressive, and more creative in their fight against that cold or flu virus. We want our leukotrienes out there protecting us from illness.

The problem with leukotrienes is not so much what they do but where they do it. You don't want leukotrienes triggering a very messy immune reaction inside the walls of your arteries. That process begins when the artery wall is violated by LDL cholesterol, homocysteine, and oxidants.

When the artery tissue is injured, the cells secrete a substance called arachidonic acid. Immune cells recognize the presence of arachidonic acid in the bloodstream like sharks recognizing blood in the water. They immediately come bounding down on the injury and search out its cause. Naturally they stumble upon the oxidized cholesterol, homocysteine, and free radicals. The immune cells gobble up (or phagocytize) these oxidized particles. As the firefight proceeds, immune cells start releasing cytokines, some of which are designed to transform monocytes into macrophages — more mature and powerful cells. Our leukotrienes call out other immune cells, and in so doing promote an even more advanced inflammatory process.

When large numbers of immune cells gather inside the walls of your arteries, they start releasing leukotrienes—lots of them. The abundance of chemical messengers overstimulates immune cells, so that more immune cells arrive on the scene. Now you've got a bunch of hyperactive immune cells, many of them producing oxidants, or free radicals, that only serve to pollute the immediate environment even more. More oxidation, more immune cells, and more leukotrienes mean more inflammation, and inflammation can weaken even a small plaque and cause it to rupture. When that happens, clotting proteins, fibrinogen, and homocysteine can combine to form a clot large enough to cause a heart attack.

Even when a clot is not formed, changes occur in the artery that lead to serious problems. Leukotrienes cause vasoconstriction, the contraction of the arteries and blood vessels, which makes them thicker and less flexible. Thick, hardened vessels cannot expand to allow more blood to flow when needed. Such a condition can lead to high blood pressure, reduction of blood flow to the heart and brain, and an increased risk of heart attack or stroke. High blood pressure itself also causes injury to arteries and sets off the inflammatory process.

All of these factors are controlled by diet. Too much fat and protein—which drive up cholesterol, homocysteine, fibrinogen, and free radicals—boost leukotrienes and promote greater inflammation. Another important behavior that boosts cholesterol, homocysteine, free radicals, and leukotrienes is cigarette smoking, which is toxic to the body in just about every way possible.

Bacteria: The Freeloader in Plaque Formation

Once you've got an open wound in the artery wall and a lot of immune activity going on, the wound becomes even bigger and more inflamed. And here come opportunistic bacteria, which are always looking for open, unprotected tissue to feed on and multiply. The bacteria enter the wound, hoping perhaps to duck under the immune system's radar—the immune system being preoccupied with all that oxidized cholesterol and homocysteine.

Where does the bacteria come from? There are always small populations of bacteria in your system, even when you're healthy. But significant bacterial infection is common among many people. People with gingivitis, or gum disease, which is created by high populations of the bacteria *Streptococcus pneumoniae*, are at a much higher risk of having heart disease. So, too, are those with ulcers, created by the bacteria *Helicobacter pyloria* and the community-acquired pneumonia caused by *Chlamydia pneumoniae*. In fact, dentists first made the connection between bacterial contamination and heart disease, when they noticed that people with gingivitis were more likely to have heart disease. When scientists studied this hypothesis, they found it to be valid. Bacteria alone cannot cause heart disease. But the more bacteria or infectious agents there are in your system—even an apparently non-life-threatening one such as gum disease—the greater your risk of heart attack and stroke. For this reason I am not surprised by the recent association between individuals receiving smallpox vaccinations and heart attacks, since our earlier experience with smallpox vaccination has been in younger people who should have less heart disease and not with individuals with significant risk factors for underlying heart disease.

Interestingly, people with healthy arteries do not have bacteria in their artery tissue. The reason? There's no entry wound in the artery wall for bacteria to sneak in and take advantage of.

No sooner have bacteria set up housekeeping in your artery tissue than your immune system recognizes their presence. The first member of your defenses to spot the bacteria is complement, an immune-system protein whose purpose is to keep down the population of bacteria and viruses in your system. As described earlier, this protein's rather interesting way of dealing with bacteria is to poke holes in their cell membranes. This is usually effective, and complement can handle small populations of bacteria just fine, but if the streptococcus, chlamydia, or helicobacter are too numerous, complement needs help. One of the ways it calls out the cavalry is by popping little holes into healthy tissue cells. In other words, it makes a mess of your artery. As more holes are poked into artery tissue, more inflammation is created.

The presence of additional wounds in the artery is the signal calling more advanced immune cells, which now arrive in much greater numbers. At this point, oxidized LDL cholesterol, homocysteine, free radicals, fibrinogen, Lp(a), growth factors, and whole hordes of immune cells and complement are all doing combat in the artery wall. The immune cells secrete more cytokines, including many more inflammatory leukotrienes. The net effect is even more inflammation, which means more unstable plaques, more vasoconstriction, and more clot formation. In short, a greater chance of heart attack.

Interestingly, certain foods will increase the presence of these inflammatory leukotrienes, the most notable of which are cow's-milk products. Numerous studies have shown that in sensitive people, milk proteins can trigger production of inflammatory cytokines (tumor necrosis factor, interleukin-2 and -5, and leukotriene B4). This is especially the case in children who have a milk sensitivity, and in people who suffer from rheumatoid arthritis. Studies have show that elimination of milk products significantly reduces inflammation throughout the bodies of people who have a milk sensitivity.

An Antibiotic Treatment for Heart Disease

The presence of bacteria as a factor in heart disease is a recent discovery; I have been treating it effectively as an element in the Fleming Program for several years now by using a mild antibiotic regimen: 500 mg of Biaxin, taken twice a day, for 14 days. This has proved to be an effective approach to reducing bacteria and leukotriene levels. Your doctor can determine whether you have high bacterial levels, and the test for your C-reactive protein levels is important because it indicates the presence of inflammation and possible infection. SPECT tests done before and after treatment have shown that after two weeks of treatment the patient often experiences significantly improved blood flow to the heart. The following case history is but one of many such examples.

Peter's Story

Peter had all the signs of an inflammatory process that was triggered in part by the presence of bacteria. He had had a heart attack in January 2002 and was referred to me two months later. His previous angiograms had revealed that all of his coronary arteries were occluded by 80 percent or more. Ironically, his cholesterol level wasn't all that bad, just under 170 mg/dL, and neither were his triglycerides. But he obviously had heart disease, and the bigger picture had to be looked at.

Sure enough, his tests revealed that his blood was highly viscous and prone to clot formation. His doctors wanted to put him on a blood thinner, but Peter had had colon cancer, which ruled out any use of anticoagulants. Such drugs could increase his risk of bleeding.

No, the clotting had to be dealt with in other ways—specifically, diet and exercise habits. Peter's homocysteine and leukotriene levels were elevated. Both of these risk factors promote blood clotting and increase blood viscosity.

They also increase inflammation. Therefore, it came as no surprise to me that his C-reactive protein was elevated.

This does not necessarily imply a bacterial infection, because you can have inflammation without bacteria. Another test, however, was revealing: Peter's acute-phase antibodies were four times greater than normal. Acute-phase antibodies are produced by immune cells called B cells, which make antibodies to fight bacterial infection. The antibodies revealed the presence of chlamydia, and so I put him on a two-week regimen of Biaxin. Sure enough, two weeks later, Peter's angina pain had completely disappeared, and blood flow to his heart had improved substantially.

Peter made steady improvement on the diet and continues to show improvement in all of his risk factors. He has not had chest pain in more than a year.

How to Reduce Leukotriene Levels and Inflammation

The key to getting leukotriene levels to fall is to protect the arteries from injury. Without injury to arteries, there is no release of arachidonic acid and no attraction of immune cells that produce leukotrienes. The main factors that wound the artery wall are blood cholesterol, homocysteine, and oxidants. The way to reduce all of these almost overnight is fairly simple:

- Reduce fat intake.
- Eliminate animal proteins until your numbers are well inside the safe range.
- Eat only vegetables and fruits, which will rapidly lower blood cholesterol and increase folic acid, vitamin B_6, and antioxidants.
- Take a multivitamin that includes antioxidants and vitamin B_{12}, which also lower cholesterol and homocysteine levels. When this is necessary, I usually prescribe Foltx, a supplement that provides folic acid and vitamins B_6 and B_{12}.

In addition, certain foods can directly lower leukotriene and other inflammatory cytokine levels. The following are especially powerful at lowering these inflammatory chemical messengers:

Ginger Root

Ginger (*Zingiber officinale*), a common root, has been shown to reduce inflammation and lower leukotriene levels. Studies have shown that it can be effective at reducing the pain of arthritis, an inflammatory illness, and can also reduce platelet aggregation and improve blood circulation. Ginger is typically grated and added to soups, stews, and vegetable medleys. It can also be grated fresh and added to vegetables.

Turmeric

A relative of the ginger root, turmeric (*Curcuma longa*) contains the active ingredient curcumin, which is a highly potent antioxidant. It has been shown to reduce inflammation and to lower leukotrienes. Studies have shown that curcumin inhibits platelet aggregation. Researchers at the M. D. Anderson Cancer Center in Houston have found that curcumin interferes with the chemical chain of events inside the cell that would otherwise lead to malignancy. Scientists in Israel have reported that people who regularly consume turmeric experience lower rates of bladder and prostate cancers. Turmeric, a common spice, is traditionally added to curry dishes to give them their familiar color and flavor. It can be used in a wide variety of dishes.

Nettle

Nettle (*Urtica urens*), a plant that has been used medicinally for centuries in Native American cultures, has been found to suppress inflammatory cytokines, including interleukin-1b and tumor necrosis factor. Human studies have found that nettle reduces inflammation, pain, and other symptoms in people with rheumatoid arthritis. Researchers have reported that nettle is as effective at reducing inflammation as nonsteroidal anti-inflammatory drugs, but does not have these medications' side effects. Doctors in Germany have long used nettle to treat a wide variety of inflammatory disorders, including arthritis. Typically, it is taken as a tincture (a solution preserved in alcohol that can be added as drops to water, juice, or tea) or as a dried herb that is steeped in water to make a tea.

Flaxseed and Other Sources
of Essential Fatty Acids

Just as saturated fats and trans-fats boost cholesterol and set the whole inflammatory cascade in motion, a certain type of essential fatty acid, omega-3 fats, reduces inflammation, protects against free radical damage, and protects the heart. Studies show that omega-3 fats reduce the inflammatory cytokines, including leukotrienes; they also strengthen the immune system and reduce the risk of cancer. Omega-3 fats are found in most plant foods, especially grains, vegetables, beans, walnuts, pumpkin seeds, and edible seaweeds. They are also abundant in flaxseed, cod, flounder, scrod, haddock, halibut, and salmon.

Many people today, especially those with rheumatoid arthritis, are taking fish oils as a supplement. The problem with taking fish oils is twofold. First, fish oils very quickly break down, oxidize, and become rancid in your tissues. Once that happens, they release hordes of free radicals, thus resulting in exactly the opposite effect that you took them for in the first place. The second problem with fish oil is that you've got to consume enormous amounts of it to make much of a difference on your immune system. Whenever you consume oil, you're consuming fat. That means that you're consuming lots of calories, and excess calories trigger the inflammatory process, which is another way that fish oils backfire on you. My advice: avoid fish oils at all costs. Eat vegetables, beans, and grains, and use crushed and roasted flaxseeds on your breakfast cereal as a condiment. You'll get plenty of omega-3s, along with an abundance of powerful immune boosters, cancer fighters, and free-radical scavengers.

We desperately need more omega-3 fats in our diet. Most Americans consume an overabundance of omega-6 fatty acids,

> **REVERSING HEART DISEASE ON THE FLEMING PROGRAM: STEPS 9, 10, AND 11**
>
> **Step 9:** Lower leukotrienes by reducing fat and protein in the diet to below 9.8 pg/mL.
>
> **Step 10:** Reduce complement by reducing overall inflammation and bacterial levels.
>
> **Step 11:** Reduce bacterial levels by asking your doctor to prescribe a low-dose antibiotic, such as 500 mg of Biaxin, to be taken twice a day for a short duration, such as 14 days.
>
> *

which suppress the immune system and promote cancer. Omega-6 fats are found in corn oil, safflower oil, sunflower oil, cottonseed oil, and most processed foods. Ideally, we should be getting an equal amount of omega-3s and omega-6s, but most people get only 1 omega-3 fatty acid for every 20 omega-6s.

These four plant-based substances—ginger, turmeric, nettle, and flaxseed—can be added to your diet and can be highly effective at reducing inflammation and leukotrienes. They are inexpensive plant-based forms of medicine that add spice and flavor to your foods while they help you avoid a heart attack or stroke. Not a bad way to keep your heart healthy.

Protect Your Arteries

BILL, 37, A HUSBAND AND THE FATHER of three, weighed 300 pounds and experienced shortness of breath and crushing chest pain whenever he exerted himself. His chest pain was so bad that it would sometimes cause him to vomit. In addition to these symptoms, Bill's blood cholesterol level was 250 mg/dL, and his triglyceride level was 340 mg/dL.

Bill's doctors performed an angiogram and an echocardiogram on his heart. An angiogram involves the injection of a contrast solution into the coronary arteries. An X-ray machine is then used to determine if there is atherosclerotic plaque protruding from the inside of the artery walls. An echocardiogram is a test that bounces sound waves off the heart and back onto a monitor, which then creates an accurate picture of the heart and its inner workings.

After these and other tests, Bill's doctors pronounced him well. He was fine, they told him. No heart disease. As for the pain, it was a mystery. Maybe it was indigestion or stress-related. Go home and rest. Take some time off. Learn to relax, they said.

Bill came to me in October 2000. I ran my standard battery of tests on him: blood cholesterol, homocysteine, fibrinogen, C-reactive protein, Lp(a), and growth factors. All of them were abnormally high. I then performed a SPECT test on his heart; it revealed extensive coronary heart disease.

"How could my doctors tell me that I didn't have heart disease?" Bill asked me.

"Angiograms can detect the plaques that grow into the opening of the artery, called the lumen," I said. "They can't see diseased artery tissue. At first, atherosclerosis grows down into the artery wall. It isn't until much later in the disease process that the plaques grow into the pathway of the artery. That means that angiograms can't see the disease if it's in the artery tissue but not in the lumen. That doesn't mean that you don't have diseased arteries. What's worse, it doesn't mean you can't have a heart attack. Small plaques can erupt and cause a blood clot that's large enough to bring on a heart attack or a stroke. Most people die from heart attacks that are caused by plaques that are relatively small," I said.

Even before such plaques trigger a heart attack, they can sometimes cause chest pain. Chest pain is caused by regional differences in blood and oxygen flow to the heart. Arteries have to expand when the heart is forced to work harder. But diseased arteries expand to very different degrees. One artery may be able to expand and allow the flow of as much as 70 percent of the blood needed by the heart under exertion. Another may be much more diseased and constricted and may allow only 30 percent of the blood needed by the heart. All of which means that one part of the heart is getting a lot more blood and oxygen than another. Oxygen starvation in a heart muscle very often causes chest pain.

I placed Bill on a cholesterol-lowering medication and a nitroglycerine drug, which helped relieve his chest pain. He also adopted Phase 1 of the Fleming Program. The cholesterol-lowering medication and nitroglycerine brought about an immediate relief in his symptoms. Meanwhile, the Phase 1 diet changed his health fundamentally. He lost 70 pounds in three months. His cholesterol dropped to 170 mg/dL, and his triglycerides to below 150 mg/dL. His other tests—homocysteine, fibrinogen, C-reactive protein, and Lp(a)—all fell into the normal ranges as well. I was delighted, to say the least.

In the months that followed, Bill continued to lose weight and eventually got down to about 200 pounds. I was also able to gradually wean him of his medication. As far as I was concerned, he had made a complete recovery from heart disease.

Doctors or Plumbers?

Our old understanding of heart disease led us astray in many ways. The first, and perhaps most important, was to view arteries as something like copper pipes. That understanding encouraged doctors to treat the illness as if they were plumbers. Beware of doctors when they think like plumbers! Three of the most common forms of treatment for coronary heart disease are based on the plumber mentality. Balloon angioplasty essentially is an attempt to crush the obstruction into the blood vessel and thereby open the pathway so that more blood can flow. A second treatment, the implantation of a stent, involves the insertion of a small tube inside the artery. The stent crushes the plaque and acts as an inner lining, or a sleeve, whose purpose is to keep the artery open. Finally, coronary bypass surgery requires the rerouting of plumbing around the old, obstructed pipes and replacing them with clear pipes.

Unfortunately, none of these methods provides a long-term solution, because arteries are not metal pipes. Arteries are living tissue. When they are damaged, they attempt to heal themselves by triggering an immune reaction. That immune reaction creates an inflammatory process that will eventually create a plaque and a blood clot. The more injuries, the greater the likelihood of clots. If a person's diet raises blood cholesterol, homocysteine, fibrinogen, and Lp(a), to name just a few of the threatening factors, the injuries will be numerous and the blood clots potentially life-threatening. It's that simple.

In the cases of balloon angioplasty and the insertion of a stent, the artery is injured as a consequence of the treatments. In both cases, the treatments trigger inflammatory processes that eventually produce new plaques and blot clots. Furthermore these interventions, and the angiogram as well, involve inserting a catheter into a blood vessel, and this procedure brings its own set of hazards. As for bypass surgery, the clear arteries soon become occluded just like the old ones, unless you adopt a diet that protects the arteries from inflammation.

These are all obvious examples of the plumber mentality in action. Furthermore, this old way of approaching heart disease has led to our dependence upon coronary angiograms as a leading method of diagnosis. Angiograms, like angioplasty, stents, and bypasses, are also based on the plumber approach.

Essentially, angiograms tell us whether or not the pipes are visibly blocked. According to this way of seeing things, you've either got a hairball and a bar of soap stuck in your plumbing, or your pipes are clear. If you've got the hairball and the soap, you've got heart disease. If your pipes appear clear, you're free of illness. Unfortunately, heart disease is more complicated than that. The illness actually arises within the wall of the artery, which means that you may have a life-threatening disease long before you develop a hairball in your coronary vessel that is visible by means of angiography.

That was the case with Bill. He had all the factors that injure arteries and cause blood clots: elevated cholesterol, homocysteine, triglycerides, fibrinogen, C-RP, and Lp(a). When viewed from the new understanding of heart disease as an inflammatory illness, Bill was clearly in trouble. In addition to everything else, his C-reactive protein level was elevated, which indicated that he did, in fact, suffer from high levels of inflammation. When those clues were coupled with his crushing chest pain, the diagnosis should have been a no-brainer. Heart disease, pure and simple. But the angiogram came back negative, meaning there was no disease visible to the X-ray machine. Because we have become so dependent upon angiograms and so locked into the plumber mentality, a single element in the picture can lead to an incorrect, potentially fatal, diagnosis. Fortunately, Bill pursued the matter until he got the right diagnosis, and the right treatment for his illness.

Medical Consequences of the Plumber Mentality

Just because you have a clear angiogram does not mean you do not have heart disease. In fact, angiograms can only see advanced disease, which, ironically, may not even be the most dangerous, for small plaques are often the most unstable and most vulnerable to rupture and clot formation. Those are the ones that kill people.

The problem is that our new knowledge hasn't saturated medicine and the public's understanding sufficiently to change the way most cardiologists diagnose and treat this illness. We are still relying primarily on angiograms to determine whether or not a person has coronary atherosclerosis. Unfortunately, the plumber mentality remains in force, and balloon angioplasty and stents remain leading forms of treatment.

Angioplasty: Crushing Your Arteries

Each year, more than 900,000 balloon angioplasties are performed in the United States, according to the American Heart Association. The primary reasons behind angioplasty are debilitating angina pectoris (chest pain) and proven occlusion, or blockage, of one or more coronary arteries. Under these conditions, a balloon catheter is utilized to open the artery to allow more blood to flow to the heart.

The catheter is passed through the artery until it reaches the diseased area; then the balloon is expanded within the blood vessel, and the plaque is crushed into the artery tissue. Bits of the debris are freed from the plaque and allowed to float downstream, where they can become lodged in places where the artery narrows, or where other plaques have formed and partially block blood flow. They can also flow into the heart itself. Dr. Eric Topol, head of cardiology at the Cleveland Clinic, reported in March 2000 that these tiny particles that float downstream following angioplasty can and do cause small heart attacks. These small heart attacks kill part of the heart tissue, reduce the heart's overall function, and make the person more vulnerable to a fatal heart attack. We know that angioplasty can cause a heart attack, says Topol, because of the highly detailed and abundant information about the heart provided by nuclear imaging (SPECT tests).

Other problems arise from balloon angioplasty. When the balloon expands and crushes the plaque, growth factors are released, which can promote the formation of a clot and cause the artery to contract, thus making it more narrow and decreasing blood flow to the heart. There is a 1 in 1,000 chance of having a heart attack or a stroke on the day you undergo cardiac catheterization for either balloon angioplasty or an angiogram.

I remember being a young doctor and working with an attending physician while he administered an angiogram to a middle-aged woman. The catheter had been threaded through the aorta, the major artery that runs down the center of the body, and into the coronary artery. Unbeknownst to us, the catheter had ruptured the aorta and was causing internal bleeding. The woman began to scream, "I'm in pain, I'm in pain." The attending physician instructed that she be given more nubain, a narcotic pain reliever, but the pain continued. It was most acute, she said, in her back. We did an ultrasound test and discovered that the blood had pooled in her abdomen and around her kidneys. Had we not done that test, and acted quickly once we had the results, that woman might have died. The experience, which occurred early in my medical training, taught me how dangerous catheterization can be. We should not only utilize catheterization with great caution but also recognize its limitations.

Balloon angioplasty has never been shown to save lives or extend life, though it has killed a minority of those who undergo the operation. Its only value is to relieve chest pain, something that can be accomplished with dietary change and drug treatment.

Most of these same things can be said about the insertion of a stent. A stent attempts to force the artery to remain open, but, like angioplasty, it triggers an inflammatory reaction that eventually creates a new plaque and closure of the artery. The only reason to insert a stent is to temporarily relieve chest pain, yet Vice President Richard Cheney had a stent implanted in one of his coronary arteries and soon suffered angina pain nonetheless.

Bypass Surgery: Another Short-Term Fix

Bypass surgery is done most often for two reasons: to relieve disabling chest pain and to extend life. Bypass surgery is only supposed to be done after the heart has failed to respond adequately to drug treatment. The operation involves removing one or more arteries from other places in the body—usually the mammary artery in the chest or the saphenous vein in the leg—and using those healthy, clean vessels to reroute blood around one or more of the occluded arteries that lead from the aorta to the heart.

CONDITIONS FOR PERFORMING BYPASS SURGERY

Doctors are supposed to perform a bypass operation only when a patient suffers from one or more of the following conditions:

1. *The heart muscle has been significantly weakened.* Doctors determine the strength of the heart by measuring the ability of the left ventricle, the heart's lower left chamber, to push out blood. That ability is referred to as the "ejection fraction." A normal, healthy heart can push out more than

50 percent of the blood that enters the left ventricle (the rest stays in the ventricle). But if the heart cannot "eject" half of the blood that enters, or can eject as little as 35 percent, it means that the heart has been severely weakened and that the person is a candidate for bypass surgery. However, if the patient's ejection fraction is below 30 percent, the heart may be too weak to withstand the operation, and there is an increased risk of losing the patient during the surgery.

Studies have shown that people with ejection fractions between 50 and 35 percent who undergo bypass surgery tend to live longer than those who do not have the surgery.

2. *The left main coronary artery is blocked.* The left main coronary artery, which is the largest of the vessels feeding the heart, divides into two branches: the left anterior descending (LAD), which runs down the center of the heart; and the circumflex branch (LCx), on the left side of the heart. The other main artery is the right coronary (RCA) artery, which branches into the marginal and posterior descending branches and supplies blood to the right side of the heart. From these three large vessels (LAD, LCx, RCA) flow many smaller arteries that also nourish the heart muscle. Smaller vessels can develop to provide blood flow to areas of the heart where disease in the larger arteries cannot supply adequate oxygen and nutrients. These are called collaterals, or collateral arteries. The left main is like a big river that feeds many smaller rivers. If that gets blocked, you're in real trouble. Studies show that people whose left main coronary artery is more than 70 percent blocked do live longer if they undergo the surgery.

3. *All three main coronary arteries (the right coronary vessel, the left anterior descending, and the circumflex vessel) are significantly narrowed.* This is usually referred to as "triple vessel disease." When this condition occurs, coupled with a low ejection fraction, it's probably a good idea to have the surgery, and doctors typically recommend it.

4. *The left anterior descending artery is more than 90 percent narrowed.* Studies have shown that people with normal ejection fractions and significant closure of the left anterior descending who have the surgery do not live any longer than those who don't.

Based on the four scenarios above, the following conclusions can be drawn: Researchers have found that people who have the first two symptoms and have the surgery live longer than those who don't have the operation. People who have the third condition—narrowing of all three main coronary arteries—coupled with low ejection fractions have been found to live longer if they have undergone bypass surgery.

THE DANGERS OF THE BYPASS

More than 600,000 bypass operations take place worldwide each year. So routine has the operation become that many people today consider it a part of the aging process. Few people realize that there are some very serious side effects. Among the most troubling of these is the fact that nearly everyone who undergoes a bypass operation experiences some degree of brain damage, which is permanent for 15 to 44 percent of those people. People report experiencing significant memory loss, sleep disturbances, loss of mental acuity, mood swings, and depression.

Why does such brain damage occur? In order for the surgery to be performed, a person's heart is almost stopped (beating only a few times each minute) and a heart-lung machine is used to pump and circulate the blood throughout the body. While in the machine, the blood can be poisoned by an array of toxic substances, gases, globules of fat, bits of debris, and even plastic particles, all of which eventually make their way to the brain, where they can do significant damage.

The operation itself can be fatal. Ten percent of those who undergo a bypass surgery die during the procedure or immediately afterward. Thirteen percent experience serious side effects, including heart attacks, strokes, kidney failure, internal bleeding, and infection.

There are people for whom bypass surgery is necessary. However, unless you meet the criteria outlined above, avoid bypass surgery. Instead, adopt the Fleming Phase 1 program and follow it to the letter. Chest pain is the primary reason that bypass surgery is done. Angina pain can be relieved through dietary change alone. That means that the right dietary regimen can make bypass surgery unnecessary.

How to Get Effective Treatment

If you go to see your doctor because you suspect you have a heart problem, the first two questions that you need to get answered are these:

1. Do you have a problem?
2. What is the cause? Which of the 12 risk factors are most out of balance and in need of correction?

These two questions should guide doctor and patient in both diagnostic and treatment procedures.

Thorough Testing for a Reliable Diagnosis

An angiogram cannot tell us definitively if you have a problem. It misses too much to tell us for certain whether you suffer from heart disease.

As I see things, testing must be very thorough if we are to correctly diagnose heart disease and its cause. When we have the answers to those two questions, we can treat your disease effectively. Here's what I do to test for heart disease.

When someone arrives in my office and shows signs of a possible heart problem, we schedule three days of extensive testing.

DAY 1

A Personal History: Looking for Signs of Disease A personal history includes the entire medical history, and also focuses on the primary risk factors for heart disease:

- *Age.* The risk of heart disease increases for both men and women as they age.
- *Family history.* People do have hereditary genetic predispositions to heart disease and other illnesses. Nonhereditary factors also tend to run in families, like the diets that give rise to the illness. I contend that improper diet makes us more vulnerable to the illnesses for which we have a hereditary genetic weakness.
- *Sex.* Men have higher rates of heart disease in their thirties, forties, and fifties than women, but after menopause the incidence among women

pulls equal to that of men, and then exceeds it. Thus, sex, age, and menopausal status are important risk factors.

- *Tobacco use.* Cigarette smoking exacerbates all other risk factors that lead to atherosclerosis and coronary heart disease. It is a major risk factor for the illness.

- *Blood pressure.* High blood pressure injures arteries and triggers the inflammatory process. People with hypertension have much higher rates of heart attacks, strokes, and kidney disease than people who do not have high blood pressure.

- *Weight.* Weight gain, even when it's relatively minor, increases inflammation and the risk of heart disease. Obese people have more than four times the risk of heart attack of people who are at their ideal weight.

- *Diabetes.* Diabetes is an inflammatory illness. Consequently, people with diabetes have much higher risk of dying from heart disease than those who do not have the illness.

- *Exercise patterns.* Sedentary lifestyles promote inflammation and numerous other risk factors for heart disease, including triglycerides, cholesterol, fibrinogen, and weight.

- *Chest pain.* Angina pectoris is a symptom of insufficient blood flow to the heart. The resultant lack of oxygen causes pain. It's a sign of significant atherosclerosis and indicates a high risk of heart attack.

- *Abnormal changes in heart rhythm.* These include irregular beating (dysrhythmia), rapid beating (tachycardia), or fluttering (an irregular beating called *ventricular fibrillation*). All irregularities suggest a weakened heart and an acute vulnerability to heart attack. (*Arrhythmia*, the term most people use when they mean *dysrhythmia*, actually means the absence of a heartbeat.)

A person who has one or more of these risk factors is at risk for heart disease. At that point, further testing is needed to find out how extensive the disease is, and which of the 12 risk factors I have described are imbalanced.

Once I have completed a physical examination and taken a personal history, I begin my testing.

Echocardiogram: A First Look at the Heart   Usually the first test I do is an echocardiogram, a noninvasive test that bounces sound waves off the heart and back onto a monitor, which can then give us an accurate picture of the heart. An echocardiogram can tell us the size of heart and the heart's wall motion, that is, whether it is flexible or stiff, or excessively thick. These signs may indicate deficient blood flow or scar tissue from a previous heart attack. An echocardiogram can also tell us how well the heart valves are functioning, whether the heart is swollen, how well the chambers are working, whether the heart has been damaged by a previous heart attack, and whether there is fluid in the pericardium, the sack that surrounds the heart, which may be a sign of heart failure.

Doppler Ultrasound Scan of the Carotid Artery Doppler ultrasonography is a non-invasive test in which a handheld device is placed over an artery and sends high-frequency sound waves into the artery. These sound waves are bounced off the red blood cells and any obstructions that may be inside the artery. This information is sent back to a monitoring device, providing an accurate reading of how well the blood is circulating inside an artery, whether there are any obstructions within the vessel, and whether there are any abnormalities in the flow of blood through the artery. When applied to the carotid artery, Doppler ultrasonography can tell us, for example, the degree of atherosclerosis in the vessel and whether there is insufficient blood flowing to the brain.

Ankle Brachial Index A noninvasive test in which a device, called a Doppler ultrasound, is applied to the ankle and senses whether there is decreased blood flow in the legs or any sign of peripheral vascular disease.

Ultrasound Test of Aorta The aorta, the body's largest artery, arises from the left ventricle and runs like the trunk of a tree down the center of the body. From its branches spring the arteries that flow to many of the body's organs, such as the spleen, kidneys, and liver. As with the carotid Doppler test, an ultrasound device is used to detect the degree of blood flow through the aorta and to determine whether there is significant blockage from atherosclerosis or clots. It can also tell if there is weakness (aneurysm) in the wall of the artery.

Blood Panel Once these noninvasive tests have been done, I run a complete blood panel on the patient—an analysis of all the important components of the blood. I ask the person not to eat breakfast on the day I will draw the blood sample because the results of the many individual tests are most accurate after a short "fast." Included in the blood panel are the following tests.

Total blood cholesterol. This is the most important of all the blood cholesterol tests. An ideal blood cholesterol level is less than 150 mg/dL. Anything above 180 mg/dL is a risk, and that risk increases dramatically above 200 mg/dL.

LDL cholesterol. The second most important cholesterol test measures low-density lipoproteins. LDL is the most toxic form of cholesterol and the one that most aggressively promotes atherosclerosis. LDL cholesterol should be less than 100 mg/dL and preferably less than 70 mg/dL.

HDL cholesterol. High-density lipoproteins offer limited protection against heart disease. If your total cholesterol is high, however, don't look to HDL to save you. The HDL level ideally should be 50 mg/dL, but if your total cholesterol level is around 150, don't worry if your HDL falls between 30 and 50. Talk to your doctor if it is lower than 30 mg/dL.

Triglycerides. A percentage of blood fats, or triglycerides, becomes LDL cholesterol. Triglycerides also reduce circulation to cells and organs. They are a risk factor for heart disease. Don't let your triglycerides get any higher than 150 mg/dL.

Fasting glucose. This tests indicates whether a person is diabetic. A normal level is below 109 mg/dL, but I prefer to see it under 100 mg/dL.

Insulin levels. High insulin is a risk factor for weight gain, diabetes, heart disease, and cancer. An ideal range is 5 to 27 μIU/mL.

Homocysteine. A normal homocysteine level is 4 to 12 μmol/L, but I prefer to see it at 10 μmol/L or lower.

Fibrinogen. Normal fibrinogen ranges from 200 to 400 mg/dL, but most doctors like to see fibrinogen levels below 350 mg/dL.

Lipoprotein (a). A healthy Lp(a) is less than 30 mg/dL. Anything above 30 indicates a liver that is distressed by numerous dietary factors and very likely triggering high degrees of inflammation.

C-reactive protein. Most labs state that a normal C-RP level is anything below 0.5 mg/dL.

Liver-function tests. AST (aspartate transaminase) is produced in the liver and is essential to energy production. The normal range is 0 to 36 international units per liter (IU/L) of blood. I also check ALT (alanine transaminase, formerly SGPT), which has a normal range of 0 to 40 IU/L. These tests reveal a great deal about liver function, which is important in the production of inflammation and the possible presence of cancer.

Kidney function. Levels of BUN (blood urea nitrogen) and sCr (serum creatinine) indicate the state of kidney function. Normal BUN is 7 to 21 mg/dL. Values above that range indicate possible kidney disorder, GI bleeding, stress, and the presence of certain drugs in the system. Decreased BUN can reflect starvation, liver failure, kidney disease, and pregnancy. The normal sCr range is 0.7 to 1.3 mg/dL. Anything above that suggests kidney disease, excessive meat intake, and the presence of certain drugs.

Interleukin-6. Normal is less than 9.8 picograms per milliliter (pg/ml). When interleukin-6 goes above those levels, you've got strong evidence for an inflammatory reaction, very likely from the risk factors for heart disease, excess milk consumption, milk allergy, as well as from bacterial infection.

After taking a personal history, doing the noninvasive tests, and drawing blood for the blood panel, I allow the person to rest and then I send him/her home. The tests continue the following day.

DAY 2

On day 2, I do a SPECT cardiac nuclear image study of the heart (see p. 23). The nuclear study of the heart has three parts: a resting study of the entire heart; a "stress" study; and an anterior, or frontal, examination of the heart and thymus gland. The thymus undergoes changes when the body is infiltrated by high levels of bacteria. I look at the thymus to determine if there is bacterial infection in the body; if present, this increases the likelihood of atherosclerosis and clot formation.

To perform a SPECT test, a small quantity of radioactive substance (containing isotopes) is injected into a vein in the arm. The material travels to the heart and is absorbed by the living tissue of the heart and the coronary arteries. The SPECT camera is positioned around the person to get views of every angle of the heart.

As described in chapter 2, a SPECT cardiac image reveals the condition of the heart all its arteries—the inner lining of the heart, its core (the endocardium), and all of the artery tissue. An angiogram can only tell you the conditions inside the arteries' pathway, or lumen, and the interior of the heart chambers, but not the artery tissue itself or the inner tissues of the heart. Heart attacks tend to occur deep inside the heart, at points farthest away from the blood supply—those are the places that get deprived of oxygen and end up dying.

A nuclear cardiac study provides a great deal of information, including the ejection fraction and the differences in regional blood flow. Also, it can provide an accurate picture of how the arteries function under stress, without actually stressing the heart with exercise.

Normally, a stress test is done by having a person walk at varying speeds on a treadmill for about 15 minutes, or until abnormalities show up in heart function. In 1 person in 10,000, that abnormality is a fatal heart attack, and nonfatal heart attacks occur far more frequently. That's the threat facing every physician who performs a stress treadmill test on a person with heart disease. On the other hand, you do want to know how much the coronary arteries can expand during exercise in order to meet the heart's needs for oxygen. Fortunately, there is a way to get around this catch-22.

A drug called high-dose dipyridamole (HDD) is used to bring about the relaxation and expansion of the arteries without forcing that reaction with exercise. During exercise, the arteries naturally expand to allow more blood and hence oxygen to flow to the heart, which it needs whenever it is forced to work harder. By opening the coronary arteries, the body provides the heart with more blood so that it can work harder without threat of a heart attack. By using a drug that triggers that expansion and monitoring the changes with the SPECT camera, I can determine how flexible the arteries are, whether they are capable of expanding to meet increased demands.

By the time the test is complete (it usually takes less than 3 hours), I have an incredibly accurate picture of the health and strength of the heart and arteries. At that point, I can make a very specific diagnosis and lay out a program for the effective treatment of the patient's heart disease.

DAY 3

On the final day of testing, I take another blood pressure reading and do another physical exam to see if there have been any changes in the person's condition since the tests were conducted. I go over with the patient all the information I have obtained—the nuclear image, the blood work, the physical examination, and the other tests. Now I can outline my treatment program. I start the person on the Fleming Program and explain any drugs to be used.

Make no mistake, medical treatment very often is essential, but it is a short-term solution designed to get the person out of the risk zone of immediate heart attack or stroke. Drugs and surgery do not cure. They offer short-term treatment that very often can save a person's life. If you view drugs and surgery as long-term cures, as so many lay and medical people do, you are in fact setting yourself up for another crisis—which usually arrives a lot sooner than you think.

Most drugs and all forms of surgery cannot provide a long-term cure because they do not deal with the underlying cause of the disease, which is inflammation. As we have seen, surgery often triggers an even greater inflammatory process, which encourages the illness. The same goes for virtually all drugs prescribed to treat heart disease. The sole exceptions to this are the NSAIDs (nonsteroidal anti-inflammatory drugs), including aspirin and ibuprofin, and the cholesterol-lowering statins, all of which may reduce inflammation. In fact, the anti-inflammatory effects of the statin drugs may, in the end, prove to be more beneficial than their ability to lower cholesterol.

Why Do We Continue Using Short-Term Approaches?

One reason that doctors and patients continue to rely on angioplasty, stents, and certain medications is that they do not want to face the fact that there is only one way to cure heart disease: significant dietary and lifestyle changes. The cause of the illness is very clear: a certain diet and lifestyle triggers an inflammatory process that results in heart attacks and strokes. The only way to cure the illness is to eliminate the foods and change the lifestyle habits that are causing the inflammation. Until medicine faces up to this immovable and rather obvious fact, doctors will not offer anything resembling a long-term solution to the leading killer in the Western world.

9

Phase 1 of the Fleming STOP INFLAMMATION NOW! Program

PICTURE YOURSELF HEALTHY, BURSTING with energy, and fully alive. Imagine that your heart is strong. Imagine that you are lean and physically fit. Picture your skin brighter, more supple, and radiating a certain healthy glow. Your limbs feel light and energetic. You sleep deeply and wake up with an enthusiasm for the day. Your eyes are clear; your mood is balanced and stable. You have a deep knowledge that your health has been restored.

These are the kinds of feelings my patients experience when they adopt the Fleming STOP INFLAMMATION NOW! Program. In fact, this program can be one of the most powerful forms of medicine you will ever experience in your life. It can change your life for the better in ways that no other form of medical care can. The reason it is able to accomplish these changes in health is because of its impact on inflammation.

The standard American diet creates a high degree of inflammation that leads to debilitating conditions and life-threatening illnesses. When you think of inflammation, think of its symptoms: heat, swelling, pain, fever, and highly unstable plaques in your arteries. These are intense symptoms that destroy the body. Before they kill, they disrupt the body and give rise to a variety of disturbing conditions that include overweight, chest pain, loss of circulation, fatigue, high insulin, high glucose, mood changes, and a pervasive discomfort with oneself.

The STOP INFLAMMATION NOW! program calls a halt to the inflammatory wars taking place throughout your body, and especially in your arteries. The program improves circulation and strengthens and supports your heart. It causes significant weight loss, boosts your immune system, increases your energy, and brings all your inflammatory markers back into normal ranges. In other words, it can give you the experience of real health, not just the remission of symptoms.

I will not attempt to fool you by saying that the changes I am about to suggest are small alterations in your lifestyle. No, the changes I'm about to recommend are radical. But that's what it takes to get your health back. Anyone who tells you that you can eat some semblance of the standard American diet and regain your health is just trying to fool you.

I strongly urge you to remain in close contact with your doctor while you follow the Fleming Program so that your doctor can follow your progress and wean you of any drugs you may be taking, including those for high cholesterol, high blood pressure, angina pectoris pain, or high blood sugar. If you practice the diet diligently, all of these blood values are likely to change for the better. Your blood pressure will also fall. It's very important that your doctor recognize your improvement and alter your medication accordingy, especially in connection with blood pressure medication. As your blood pressure falls naturally, your medication will have to be reduced in order to avoid creating a dangerously low blood pressure that could affect your heart. Allow your doctor to monitor your progress and make the necessary changes in your medication regime.

The STOP INFLAMMATION NOW! diet consists of Phase 1 and Phase 2. There is also a transition phase, which I call Phase 1a. In this chapter, I provide an in-depth look at Phase 1 and Phase 1a. In the next chapter, we look at Phase 2.

We begin with an overview of Phase 1, after which I provide an in-depth look at the foods in the regimen.

Phase 1: An Overview

On Phase 1 you eat an enormous array of vegetables and fruits. You also take a multivitamin. Though everyone knows what's in the fruit category, I do provide a comprehensive list below. People aren't always so sure about what's included in the vegetable group. Are potatoes a vegetable? Are beans and bean products considered vegetables? The answer to both questions is yes. Potatoes (tubers) and dried beans and peas (legumes) are both vegetables.

The Fleming Pyramid gives the number of servings of fruits and vegetables that you should eat each day. Initially you may be surprised by the number of servings of fruits and vegetables that are recommended, but I assure you that you will easily achieve similar numbers to these. Serving sizes are not hard and fast. A single apple is one serving of fruit. A small serving of broccoli and carrots counts as two servings of vegetables. A medley of asparagus, mushrooms, and chickpeas counts as three servings of vegetables. The menu plans in chapter 13 list three meals a day, but I encourage you to eat small meals of fruits and vegetables between meals as well. That means that it's possible to eat five or six meals a day.

Phase 1 Foods

Phase 1 includes the following foods. As you will see, some foods fall into more than one category.

Vegetables

GREEN AND LEAFY VEGETABLES

Eat eight servings per day of green and leafy vegetables, including asparagus, broccoli, cabbage, celery, chives, collard greens, kale, leeks, mustard greens, romaine lettuce, scallions, spinach, and watercress. These are goldmines of nutrition, antioxidants, and phytochemicals. They are highly anti-inflammatory and also very delicious foods.

YELLOW, ORANGE, AND RED VEGETABLES

Eat at least seven servings of yellow, red, and orange vegetables per day. In this group are beets, all forms of squash, sweet potatoes, yams, and carrots. These vegetables are pulpy and fibrous. Eat them to create feelings of full-

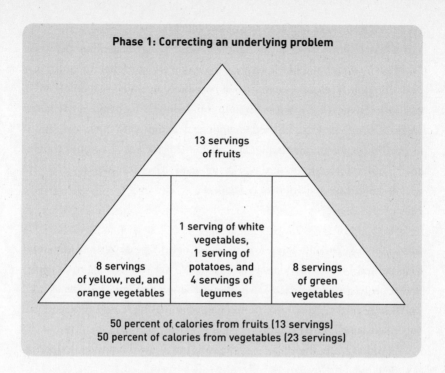

Phase 1: Correcting an underlying problem

13 servings
of fruits

8 servings
of yellow, red, and
orange vegetables

1 serving of white
vegetables,
1 serving of
potatoes, and
4 servings of
legumes

8 servings
of green
vegetables

50 percent of calories from fruits (13 servings)
50 percent of calories from vegetables (23 servings)

ness and satisfaction. Loaded with antioxidants and carotenoids, these vegetables are highly anti-inflammatory and strengthen the immune system.

WHITE VEGETABLES

Eat at least one serving per day of white vegetables such as cauliflower, daikon radish, garlic, onions, and turnips. These foods are loaded with nutrition, antioxidants, and phytochemicals. Highly anti-inflammatory, delicious, and satisfying.

TUBERS (POTATOES)

Eat at least one serving per day of potatoes, such as russet (often called Idaho potatoes), white rose (long and thin-skinned), red, and Katahdin (the most common Maine potatoes). Very satisfying and filling.

ROOT VEGETABLES

Eat at least one serving per day of a root vegetable such as carrots, burdock, lotus root, parsnips, and rutabaga. Make root stews, or root medleys. Combine squash and roots to make a sweet, filling, and highly satisfying dish.

LEGUMES (DRIED BEANS AND PEAS AND BEAN PRODUCTS)

Eat at least four servings, and as many as seven servings, of legumes per week. Lentils, chickpeas, and black, navy, and pinto beans are delicious, nutritious, and filling. This category includes bean products such as tofu, tempeh, miso, and various types of soy sauces (descriptions below), which are also delicious and satisfying. Many can be used to produce delicious soup stocks and sauces, as I will show you in this chapter and chapter 14 (recipes). Legumes contain many important nutrients and phytochemicals. They provide very powerful anti–heart disease and anticancer factors.

Fruit

Eat 13 servings per day. There is a multitude of fruit, perhaps more than most of us realize. I recommend that you eat lots of fruit—everything from apples and pears to cantaloupe and kiwis to grapes and grapefruit. Eat lots of fruit. You'll lose weight, experience more energy and lightness, and your skin will very likely appear more youthful.

As you can see, the Phase 1 regimen is not a one-dimensional, deprivation diet, but a highly varied, fully satisfying array of foods.

FLAXSEEDS AND PUMPKIN SEEDS

Eat one teaspoon of roasted and ground flaxseeds as a condiment on vegetables daily. Flaxseeds are rich in bioflavonoids, which are powerful antioxidants, and are rich in omega-3 fatty acids and other phytochemicals that are highly anti-inflammatory.

Eat three teaspoons of pumpkin seeds per week, also as a condiment on vegetables. Pumpkin seeds are rich in omega-3 fatty acids and reduce inflammation.

Daily Supplement

In addition to the recommended foods, Phase 1 also includes a daily multivitamin supplement. The supplement should include the following nutrients in dosages that are at, or near, the recommended amounts.

- Folic acid—5 mg
- Vitamin C—500 to 1,000 mg

- Vitamin E—400 to 800 international units (IU)
- Vitamin B$_6$—up to 100 mg
- Vitamin B$_{12}$—5 micrograms (μcg)
- Selenium—50 to 100 μcg

Other nutrients that can be included in the multivitamin are beta-carotene and other carotenoids, additional B vitamins, including riboflavin and thiamine, magnesium, manganese, potassium, and calcium (up to 500 mg).

Whenever possible, get food-based vitamins and minerals, which can be easier than synthetic vitamins for the body to absorb and utilize.

Beverages

On Phase 1 you may drink the following:

- *Pure, clean spring water.* Preferably without carbonation, which can upset digestion for many people. Drink six to eight large glasses a day.
- *Black and green tea.* Tea contains 20 to 45 mg of caffeine per cup, depending on how long the tea is steeped, as opposed to coffee, which contains 125 to 200 mg of caffeine, depending on how it is brewed. Avoid coffee. If you like, drink one to two cups of black or green tea per day. Tea is rich in bioflavonoids, which are powerful antioxidants (see below). If you are sensitive to caffeine, avoid caffeinated teas; drink noncaffeinated herbal teas and grain coffee.
- *Grain coffees.* Made without coffee beans or caffeine.
- *Herbal teas.*

Foods to Avoid on the Phase 1 Diet

Avoid the following pro-inflammatory foods.

- *All animal foods.* This includes red meat, pork, chicken, turkey, eggs, dairy products, and fish.
- *All oils.* This includes corn, olive, safflower, sunflower, palm kernel, coconut, and peanut oils. Oil is **liquid fat.** It will promote weight gain and inflammation. During Phase 1, we want your health to rebound quickly.

Therefore, we want to avoid all inflammatory fats, including oils. Limited amounts of certain oils are permitted during Phase 2.

- *All processed foods and flour products.* This includes rolls, muffins, pastries, bread (including whole-wheat bread). These foods are very high in calories. Many baked products contain trans-fatty acids, or hydrogenated oils, which are highly inflammatory.
- *Pasta and oatmeal.* Pasta is avoided on Phase 1, but permitted on Phase 2. Pasta, even whole-wheat pasta, is a processed food. However, both semolina durum wheat pasta and whole-wheat pasta are rich in complex carbohydrates, and neither is particularly abundant in calories, contrary to what many people believe. Pasta becomes calorically dense when oil, olives, and other fatty foods are added to the noodles. Phase 2 provides instructions on how to make your pasta less calorically dense. As for oatmeal, it is permitted on Phase 2, even though it is mildly processed. I recommend steel-cut oats, which are less processed than rolled oats. Steel-cut oats can be cooked in 25 minutes. They are crunchy and delicious.
- *Dairy products.* This includes cow's milk, cheese, butter, and yogurt. Dairy foods promote production of inflammatory cytokines, including insulin-like growth factor (IGF-1).
- *Sugar.* Includes all forms of processed sugar, including white cane sugar, brown sugar, raw sugar, maple syrup, honey, molasses, rice syrup, barley malt, and all sugar substitutes.

Do Not Eat After 7 P.M.

Most people go to sleep between 10 P.M. and midnight. If there's food in your stomach, your sleep will be disturbed. Also, after 7 P.M., the body tends to convert any calories still in the stomach into fat and triglycerides, thus increasing weight gain, cholesterol levels, and blood fats.

Comfort Foods

As we all know, people eat for reasons other than hunger. The most common other reason for eating is comfort. If you are a big comfort eater but want to lose weight and restore your health with the Phase 1 program, here are a few recommendations to help you achieve your goals.

COMFORT VEGETABLES

Eat squash and sweet vegetables every day, especially at dinner. These foods are especially sweet when cooked until they become soft and luscious. Combine sweet vegetables into a medley and cook until they become a rich and moist mixture that is very satisfying (see recipes in chapter 14). Among the sweetest vegetables are carrots, beets, parsnips, onions, sweet potatoes, yams, and squashes (acorn, butternut, delicata, Hokkaido pumpkin, Hubbard, pumpkin, yellow squash, and zucchini).

FRESH AND COOKED FRUIT

Make cooked fruit compotes. Baked apples with raisins, cooked peaches and berries, and pears and raisins are among the wide variety of fruits that can be combined to create delicious and satisfying desserts. They are also low-calorie comfort foods.

NATURAL THICKENERS

Learn to use natural thickeners such as kuzu and agar to make low-calorie fruit puddings and fruit jellies. Kuzu is a white powdered thickener that is derived from the kuzu plant, which grows wild throughout the southern United States, as well as in Asia. Dissolve two tablespoons in a cup of cold water. Meanwhile, in a saucepan, cook a variety of fruit such as apples and berries in water until the fruit is soft. Turn down the flame and add the kuzu mixture to the warm fruit and water and stir for about 5 minutes, until it thickens into a thick, rich fruit pudding. Delicious, luscious, and satisfying. Also very low in calories.

Agar is a tasteless and odorless gelatinous extract of certain seaweeds that is popular in Indonesia and much of Asia. Add it to any fruit dish that has been cooked in water and let it sit. It will thicken into a fruit aspic with the consistency of gelatin. Also very delicious and a very low-calorie dessert.

* * *

In chapter 13, I provide three weeks of menus each for Phase 1 and Phase 2. In chapter 14, you will find more than 50 recipes for delicious soups, entrées, and desserts for both Phases 1 and 2.

Rationale for Phase 1

In order to experience the most dramatic results from the Fleming Program, I urge you to adhere to Phase 1 until you have achieved the goals listed below. Phase 1 is designed to take you out of immediate danger of having a heart attack or a stroke. Recent research has shown that a low-fat, plant-based diet significantly lowers blood cholesterol, blood pressure, and the risk of heart attack in less than three weeks, even in men who are obese. Phase 1 of the Fleming Program can achieve these results—and more—even faster.

The Phase 1 diet is designed to achieve the following goals.

1. Reduce weight until you arrive at your ideal weight. Phase 1 is exceedingly low in calories, which means that it will cause you to lose excess weight rapidly and safely.

   Remember that in order to lose a pound a week, you must drop at least 350 to 500 calories a day from your diet. On the Phase 1 program, you will very likely reduce your calorie intake by more than 500 calories a day, which means that you will be losing at least a pound a week, and probably more.

   You can eat as many of the foods listed for the Phase 1 regimen as you like. You do not have to restrict the volume of food you eat. The foods on Phase 1 are so low in calories, and so rich in water and fiber, that you will feel full and satisfied, yet your calorie intake will fall.

2. Reduce blood cholesterol and triglycerides quickly and safely, and use up lipid and fat stores in your tissues. There's no saturated fat in the Phase 1 diet; it is low in calories and high in antioxidants and fiber. All of these factors make it a powerful approach to lowering cholesterol.

3. Restore homocysteine levels to normal and elevate your blood and cellular levels of antioxidants. The diet has no animal protein, which means it will cause methionine and homocysteine levels to fall. At the same time, Phase 1 is high in vegetables, beans, and fruit, all of which provide abundant amounts of folic acid, vitamin B_6, and antioxidants. A multivitamin provides appropriate amounts of vitamin B_{12}, as well as additional antioxidants, vitamins, and minerals. Thus, the Fleming Program is a formula for bringing down homocysteine levels. High antioxidant consumption will also reduce oxidation and result in significantly fewer injuries to the arteries.

4. Restore fibrinogen and growth factors to normal levels. Phase 1 is exceedingly low in fat, which lowers fibrinogen and reduces the tendency of the blood to clot. The diet is low in calories and contains no processed foods, so that insulin levels stay low. There are also no milk products in Phase 1. The low insulin and absence of milk products keep growth factors down, especially IGF-1.

5. Reduce leukotrienes, cytokines, and bacterial levels to normal. By lowering cholesterol, oxidation, and homocysteine, you reduce the injuries to your arteries. With fewer injuries, there are fewer cytokines produced and less inflammation. Fewer injuries to arteries also means a significant reduction of bacteria in the arteries. People with fewer injuries in their arteries have lower bacterial levels in the plaques.

6. Introduce and maintain a gentle, anti-inflammation exercise program. A nonstrenuous walking regimen is recommended (described on page 157).

7. Strengthen your immune system. The Phase 1 diet is extremely high in nutrition, antioxidants, and other immune-system boosters. It will boost immunity while lowering inflammation.

8. Dramatically increase energy levels. Phase 1 provides an abundance of complex carbohydrates, which give long-lasting energy. Its low fat content promotes weight loss and improvements in circulation, both of which tend to increase vitality and overall energy levels.

9. Restore a more youthful appearance and vigor to your body. When you lose weight, increase energy, and eat copious amounts of antioxidants, your appearance often improves significantly. Skin becomes brighter and takes on a healthier color. You feel more relaxed, more at peace with yourself. The high levels of complex carbohydrates also elevate a brain chemical called serotonin, which promotes feelings of well-being, confidence, and security. These inner feelings change the way you appear and how you interact with others. Gradually, a transformation takes place in which you become a more balanced human being. And it shows in your physical appearance and in the way you conduct yourself every day.

Phase 1 is not only a powerful approach to heart disease and other illnesses but also a way of restoring much of the beauty and vitality to your life. Let's get a closer look at Phase 1.

Phase 1: In Depth

Phase 1 begins with vegetables, which are the primary source of nutrition for all animals, including humans. Plant foods, including vegetables and fruits, are the core of the STOP INFLAMMATION NOW! program. The reason, very simply, is that they are loaded with anti-inflammatory compounds, most notably antioxidants, carotenoids, flavonoids, polyphenols, and other phytochemicals.

Plant Foods: Where the Nutrients Are

Vegetables are the primary source of minerals and vitamins in the food supply. The only reason animal foods provide any nutrition at all is because animals eat plants. It's that simple. Plants provide all but two of the essential vitamins and minerals that your body needs. And they do it in abundance. The two missing nutrients are vitamin B_{12}, which is provided by bacteria, and vitamin D, which is given to us by sunlight. I have included vitamin B_{12} in my supplement recommendations, so there's no chance of getting an inadequate supply of this vitamin. Deficiencies are rare. As for vitamin D, 20 minutes of daylight, even when under cloud cover, will give you all the vitamin D your body needs. Vitamin D is fat-soluble, which means your body stores it to ensure that there's an adequate supply on hand.

* * *

When I describe Phase 1 to my patients, they often ask me, What about my calcium needs, and what about protein? Good questions. Let's examine these two questions.

Calcium: Go to the Source

Our culture has been brainwashed into believing that the primary sources of calcium are milk and milk products. We have also been led to believe that many of us suffer from a calcium deficiency, which means we should drink more milk. In fact, we don't need milk to get calcium, and the vast majority of Americans are not consuming inadequate calcium. In fact, we eat more calcium than most of the rest of the world; our problem is that we eat too much animal protein, which causes the body to release calcium and phosphorus from bones. Excess protein results in calcium losses.

Milk contains approximately 300 mg of calcium per cup. The protein content of milk can promote calcium losses through the kidneys, which means that milk may not be an ideal source of calcium. On the other hand, a cup of cooked collard greens contains 360 mg. Other green vegetables are also rich in the mineral. In her book *The Calcium Bible*, the nutritionist Patricia Hausman, M.S., lists some of the best calcium sources.

- 1 cup of cooked kale: 210 mg
- 1 cup of cooked collard greens: 360 mg
- 1 cup of fresh cooked broccoli: 140 mg
- 1 cup of cooked bok choy: 250 mg
- 1 cup of cooked turnip greens: 200 mg
- 1 cup of cooked mustard greens: 190 mg
- 4 ounces of tofu (about the size of a deck of cards): 150 mg
- 1 cup of cooked beans: 100 mg
- A calcium supplement: If you have a concern about calcium intake, include calcium as part of your daily multivitamin-mineral supplement.

Phase 1 is so rich in green, leafy, root, and colored vegetables that you will have no trouble meeting your calcium needs.

When you have restored your health on Phase 1 and adopt Phase 2, other sources of calcium are available, including the following:

- 1 tin of sardines: 480 mg
- 3½ ounces of salmon: 290 mg
- 3½ ounces of mackerel: 300 mg
- 3½ ounces of herring: 250 mg
- 1 cup skim milk: 302 mg

Phase 2 includes three servings of skim milk per week.

The epidemic of osteoporosis that we now suffer from is not caused by a deficiency of calcium. It's caused by excess protein consumption and a host of other factors, such as cigarette smoking and the consumption of phosphates from cola and other soft drinks.

Plant foods contain all the essential minerals in abundance. That means you not only get calcium but also rich supplies of magnesium, zinc, iron, potassium, manganese, and selenium from the Fleming Program diet. This is just one of the reasons I say that vegetables are the real source of health.

Protein: More Than Enough

The great sources of protein in the plant kingdom are beans (legumes) and bean products such as tempeh and tofu. Beans provide 20 to 30 percent of their calories in protein. One hundred grams of azuki beans contain 21 mg of protein. A hundred grams of chickpeas contain 20 mg of protein; the same amount of whole lentils contain 25 mg of protein, according to the U.S. Department of Agriculture.

Like most plant foods, legumes also provide complete proteins, meaning they offer all the amino acids needed by the body. Phase 1 of the Fleming anti-inflammation diet includes legumes, but even without them you would get all the protein your body needs from other plant sources.

However, all plant foods provide protein, and they do it in optimal quantities. The World Health Organization (WHO) studied the question of human protein needs and found that we need to obtain at least 2.5 percent of our calories from protein each day to maintain health. Since the minimum may be on the low end, WHO scientists doubled that number and stated that all men, women, and children must consume at least 5 percent of their calories from protein to sustain health. Pregnant women, the WHO found, should get at least 6 percent of their calories from protein.

In fact, on a plant-based diet, it's impossible not to meet these requirements. Plant foods that have not been processed or refined derive 6 to 45 percent of their calories from protein. The following chart lists the protein content of common foods. If you ate all of the foods listed on this chart every day, you'd derive about 20 percent of your calories from protein, which is more than enough.

Beans, vegetables, and many fruits are ideal sources of protein. Plant proteins are easily assimilated by the body, and they do not increase homocysteine levels, nor will they lower blood levels of folic acid, vitamin B_6, and vitamin B_{12}. Unlike animal-food proteins, plant proteins are not associated with osteoporosis, arthritis, and many types of cancers.

Percent of Calories Derived from Protein	
Broccoli	43
Cauliflower	33
Pinto beans	24
Zucchini	17
Corn	12
Baked potato	10
Orange	9
Rice	8
Strawberries	8

The Full Spectrum of Nutrients

Not only do plants provide for all the vitamins and minerals your body needs, but they offer broad spectrums of these nutrients. That means that the chances of deficiencies are much smaller on a plant-based diet than on a diet rich in animal foods.

CRUCIFEROUS VEGETABLES

Allow me to give you a few examples of just how packed vegetables are with nutrients. Let's look at a few cruciferous vegetables such as cabbage, Brussels sprouts, and broccoli—all of which contain substances known as isothiocyamates and indoles, which have consistently been shown to protect against cancer. Indoles convert the types of estrogen that cause breast and other forms of cancer into harmless compounds. Animal studies have shown that cruciferous vegetables are especially effective at causing this protective alteration in estrogen. Other research has shown that people who eat high amounts of collard greens, another crucifer, and cabbage, have lower rates of colon and rectal cancers. Finally, cruciferous vegetables, along with many other green, yellow, and orange veggies, inhibit the production of a certain subset of prostaglandins, known as PGE2. These hormonelike substances trigger inflammation, including in the arteries. Crucifers inhibit production of PGE2, making them very anti-inflammatory.

Here are profiles of a few of the crucifers and what they contain:

Broccoli is one of those humble superfoods. A 3.5-ounce serving has 28 calories, 1,542 IU of vitamin A, about 140 mg of vitamin C, 71 mcg of folic acid, and 325 mg of potassium. Broccoli also contains vitamin B_6, beta-carotene, manganese, protein, and complex carbohydrates. In addition, it's a potent cancer-fighter. Broccoli contains a rich supply of a chemical called sulforanphane, which detoxifies the blood and tissues and triggers the production of cancer-preventive enzymes (*Proceedings of the National Academy of Sciences*). Studies have consistently shown that broccoli, as well as other crucifers, protect against cancer.

Brussels sprouts contain vitamin A (883 IU), vitamin B_6, beta-carotene, vitamin C (85 mg), vitamin E, folic acid, iron, manganese, and potassium.

Cabbage provides vitamin C, folic acid, and plenty of indoles.

Cauliflower contains vitamin B_6, vitamin C, folic acid, manganese, and potassium (355 mg). It is also a good supplier of indoles and other cancer-fighting substances.

Collard greens, a large, mild-tasting leafy green, are one of the richest sources of calcium and other minerals, including iron, manganese, magnesium, and copper. Collards also provide significant amounts of vitamin A, beta-carotene, vitamin B_6, vitamin C, vitamin E, and folic acid. It's also high in fiber and anti-inflammatory compounds. A wonderful food that should be eaten regularly.

Kale, like collard greens, is an amazingly nutritious leafy green vegetable loaded with nutrients, including vitamin A, vitamin B_6, vitamin C, vitamin E, beta-carotene, calcium, copper, iron, manganese, magnesium, and potassium.

Other nutritionally important crucifers include *mustard greens* and *kohlrabi*.

OTHER ANTI-INFLAMMATORY AND NUTRITIONALLY RICH VEGETABLES

Squash (genus *Cucurbita*) are rich in beta-carotene, complex carbohydrates, and potassium. Three and a half ounces of cooked butternut squash contains vitamin A (7,800 IU, the equivalent of a vitamin supplement), vitamin B_6, vitamin C, folic acid, magnesium, manganese, and potassium (352 mg). The high level of antioxidant carotenoids in squash give it wonderful anti-inflammatory properties.

Asparagus, a member of the lily family, is a delicious food that even children seem to love, and it provides only 22 calories in a 3.5-ounce serving. That little bit of asparagus gives you 119 micrograms (mcg) of folic acid,

302 mg of potassium, and plenty of fiber. Asparagus is like a vitamin A supplement, providing 897 international units (IU); it also contains significant amounts of vitamin C (33 mg).

Vegetables that are members of the *Allium* genus—*chives, garlic, leeks, onions,* and *shallots*—contain allicin and other compounds that have been shown to prevent cancer and to activate the cancer-fighting mechanisms of the body.

The carrot family includes *carrots, celery, parsley,* and *parsnips,* all of which are rich sources of carotenoids. Carrots have been shown to play an important role in the prevention of heart disease.

Vegetables in the genus *Solanum* (nightshade) include *peppers, potatoes, eggplant,* and *tomatoes.* These are rich sources of vitamin C, vitamin A, vitamin B_6, and complex carbohydrates.

Bioflavonoids: Medicinal Substances That Only Food Provides

Antioxidants are essential to protect your arteries and other tissues from oxidation, homocysteine, and inflammation. Plant foods are the most abundant sources of antioxidants, carotenoids, and phytochemicals, all of which significantly reduce inflammation.

The term "antioxidant" applies to many different types of chemicals, including a diverse group of compounds known as flavonoids, or bioflavonoids. These compounds serve as antioxidants, but they also have other health-promoting functions. Flavonoids include substances called isoflavones, which are plant hormones that protect against heart disease and common forms of cancer, including breast and prostate. Bioflavonoids are powerful inhibitors of inflammation.

The highest concentrations of bioflavonoids are found in vegetables, beans, and fruits. They are also present in black tea, green tea, and red wine. All of this points to the superiority of food over supplements. Food contains myriad substances that act on the body in very different ways. A food can provide an array of antioxidants that reduce or stop oxidation, control inflammation, and boost immune function. That same food may also provide isoflavones, or plant hormones, that protect against many forms of cancer. You can't put all of these chemicals in pill form. For one thing, we don't know all of the substances that may be active in any given food. Nor do we know how they behave synergistically to create a variety of health-promoting effects.

Even when we examine a single trait, such as antioxidation, food often does a better job than vitamin supplements. Studies have shown that 10 ounces of spinach increased blood levels of antioxidants more effectively than 1,250 mg of vitamin C taken as a supplement. When you consider that you're also getting an array of bioflavonoids with that spinach, it becomes clear that food is far superior to any supplement.

The U.S. Department of Agriculture's (USDA) Human Nutrition Research Center at Tufts University near Boston developed a scale to rate the antioxidant content of individual foods: the "oxygen radical absorbency capacity" scale, or ORAC. The following tables show the fruits and vegetables with the highest ORAC scores.

The USDA scientists found that 10 servings of fruits and vegetables per day provide 3,000 to 3,500 ORAC points—high-level protection against serious illnesses such as heart disease and cancer. On the Fleming Program Phase 1 diet, you will get many times that amount.

It's important to keep in mind that these and other fruits and vegetables contain substances that have multiple functions, in addition to their antioxidant effects. Broccoli, for example, contains a substance known as sulforanphane that has been shown to detoxify tissues and the blood and stimulate the body's cancer-fighting mechanisms. Similar compounds exist in kale, collard greens, watercress, and other green vegetables. Another example is vitamin C, one of the more powerful controllers of oxidation and inflamma-

High-ORAC Fruits

Fruit	ORAC Score
Blueberries	2,400
Blackberries	2,036
Strawberries	1,540
Raspberries	1,220
Plums	949
Oranges	750
Red grapes	739
Cherries	670
Kiwi fruit	610

High-ORAC Vegetables	
Vegetable	**ORAC Score**
Kale	1,770
Spinach	1,260
Bean sprouts	980
Brussels sprouts	980
Alfalfa sprouts	930
Broccoli flowerets	890
Beets	840
Red bell pepper	710

tion. We typically think of fruit as the primary source of C, but green and leafy vegetables are great providers of this important antioxidant.

Here are some numbers on vitamin C (from the U.S. Department of Agriculture):

* 1 cup cooked broccoli: 140 mg
* 1 cup cooked Brussels sprouts: 97 mg
* 1 cup orange juice: 97 mg
* 1 raw green pepper: 95 mg
* 1 cup fresh strawberries: 85 mg
* 1 cup cooked cauliflower: 69 mg

Carotenoids, the yellow and red pigments that color some vegetables, are powerful antioxidants, so it is no surprise that the orange, red, and yellow vegetables that contain them are good sources of antioxidants. The only source of carotenoids is plant foods.

Plants are also the best food sources of vitamin E, as the chart in chapter 5 showed. Some excellent sources of vitamin E in the Phase 1 diet are beans, flaxseeds, and pumpkin seeds.

Fiber: Essential for Health

Plant foods are the only sources of cholesterol-lowering fiber. Fiber also balances hormones (more about this in chapter 10) and binds with and eliminates many other toxins from the body. Animal foods contain no fiber. As you know, fiber is essential for the health of your digestive tract, especially your large intestine.

The short story is that, if you want to be healthy, you must eat vegetables.

Guidelines for Choosing Vegetables

Here's what I tell my patients when choosing vegetables.

- Always get the freshest vegetables you can find. Fresh vegetables have not started to decay, so they are richer in nutrients and antioxidants.
- Select organic vegetables when possible. Organic vegetables are often nutritionally richer than others and are free of pro-inflammatory chemicals such as pesticides, herbicides, and fertilizers.
- Choose the vegetables that are the richest in color. Colorful vegetables mean they are fresh and rich in nutrients, carotenoids, and bioflavonoids.
- Make leafy, green, and root vegetables the center of your diet to maximize weight loss. These foods are rich in nutrients and fiber, and are extremely low in calories.
- Eat the pulpy vegetables such as squash, potatoes, and sweet potatoes for satiety. These are highly satisfying, low-calorie comfort foods.

About Legumes and Legume Products

Not only are beans great sources of protein, they also contain significant amounts of complex carbohydrates, vitamins, minerals, and cholesterol-lowering fiber. One hundred grams of soybeans contain 226 mg of calcium, 554 mg of phosphorus, 8.4 mg of iron, and 1,677 mg of potassium, according to the USDA. All beans contain vitamin A and the B vitamins as well.

Legumes are also rich sources of substances known as isoflavones, or phytoestrogens. Plant estrogens are milder forms of the female hormone, which means they have a much less stimulating effect on sensitive tissues than the powerful estrogens produced by the body. Researchers now believe that plant estrogens may attach themselves to estrogen receptor sites on cells and block the cancer-causing estrogens produced by the body. Studies have shown that people who consume lots of phytoestrogens have significantly lower rates of breast and prostate cancer. These substances may also prevent other cancers, such as malignancies of the colon and lung. The Japanese, who eat copious amounts of bean products, especially soy foods, have 50 times the phytoestrogen and bioflavonoid levels in their blood that Westerners have. Hispanic women, who eat twice as many beans as Caucasian women, also have surprisingly low rates of breast cancer. (More on soy foods in chapter 12.) These foods are highly anti-inflammatory, thanks to their phytochemicals and antioxidants. The bioflavonoids in beans, and especially in soy foods, have been shown to prevent inflammation and heart disease as well.

Another important substance that appears to prevent cancer is an isoflavone called genistein, found in abundance in soybeans and soybean products such as tofu, tempeh, natto, tamari, and miso. Researchers have found that genistein blocks blood vessels from attaching to cancer cells and tumors, thus preventing cancer cells from getting the oxygen and nutrition they need for survival and proliferation. The attachment of blood vessels to tumors is called angiogenesis. Scientists now believe that preventing angiogenesis—or anti-angiogenesis—may be one of the most important ways of preventing cancer (*Proceedings of the National Academy of Sciences* 1993).

In fact, soybeans and soybean products are among the richest sources of anti-inflammatory, anticancer isoflavones and bioflavonoids.

Soybeans and soybean products have been shown to lower cholesterol and protect people from heart disease. The plant estrogens may be especially protective for postmenopausal women, since the phytoestrogens in soybeans may act as a mild substitute for the human estrogens that have been lost as a result of menopause.

After considering all the scientific evidence related to soy foods, the Food and Drug Administration in 1999 approved the health claim that soy foods reduce the risk of heart disease.

It's difficult to cook soybeans and serve them on their own, but there are several soybean products that are easy to prepare and will deliver an abundance of these health-enhancing substances. Here are a few soybean products that I recommend you eat regularly.

TOFU

Tofu, also known as bean curd, is essentially coagulated soy milk that's been formed into a soft block. Tofu is bursting with phytoestrogens, including genistein. It's also rich in protein and calcium (about 150 mg in a 4-oz.

serving). The Japanese eat tofu by adding grated fresh ginger (also anti-inflammatory) and one or another soybean product, namely soy sauce or tamari (described below). Both of the latter foods are fermented liquid soy condiments that are used primarily in cooking. Tofu can be added to soups, stews, noodle broths, or baked. It can also be eaten raw.

TEMPEH

Tempeh, an Indonesian food, is made from whole soybeans that have been fermented and formed into a patty. It's a wonderful source of protein, calcium, phytoestrogens, and friendly intestinal flora. Tempeh can be cut up in squares and added to soups. On Phase 2, it can be fried in sesame or olive oil and added to noodle broths.

MISO

Miso is made from a mixture of crushed soybeans and a whole grain that has been aged and fermented in salt. (Whole grain as part of miso, which is only used in small amounts in soup broths, stews, and sauces, is permissible on Phase 1.) Miso is a densely packed medium for friendly intestinal bacteria. Like other soybean products, miso is loaded with genistein and other bioflavonoids. It is most often used as a base for soup, but it can be added to noodle broths, and used as an ingredient in sauces. There are several types of miso. Each is distinguished by the grain that has been used to make it and by how long it is aged. Among the most commonly consumed misos are barley miso, rice miso, chickpea miso, and millet miso. Because miso is rich in friendly bacteria and intestinal enzymes, it is not boiled. Rather, add miso to a soup broth that has already been cooked and simmered. Boiling a soup or stew with the miso already in the broth kills the health-promoting bacteria and enzymes.

EDAMAME

Edamame is whole soybeans, still in their pods, that have been steamed and are ready to eat. Eat only the beans, not the pods. Edamame is available in the freezer sections of most supermarkets and is a great snack. Simply open the package, steam for a few minutes, and then garnish lightly with a salt substitute. These beans are rich in calcium, protein, and isoflavones.

SHOYU

Shoyu is naturally aged and fermented soy sauce. Like miso, it is a rich source of friendly bacteria and digestive enzymes. You should purchase only the shoyus that contain no artificial colors, flavors, or stimulants to fermentation. Shoyu does contain sodium—about 18 percent, which is half that of normal table salt. You can purchase low-sodium shoyu, which contains about 25 percent less sodium.

SOYMILK AND SOY CHEESE

Soymilk and soy cheeses are wonderful dairy substitutes. Soymilk is exactly what the name implies: a milk made from boiled soybeans. It contains about 150 mg of calcium per cup and is also rich in isoflavones and bioflavonoids. It contains no saturated fat and no lactose, the sugar found in milk products that causes lactose-intolerant people to suffer digestive distress.

TAMARI

Tamari is a form of shoyu that is the liquid runoff from miso production. Like shoyu, it is rich in friendly flora and digestive enzymes. Purchase low-sodium tamari.

Flaxseeds and Pumpkin Seeds

Flaxseeds are one of those foods that stands out as a nutritional anomaly. Flaxseeds contain pharmaceutical levels of isoflavones, bioflavonoids, and omega-3 fatty acids. The bioflavonoids in flaxseeds have been shown to inhibit pro-inflammatory leukotrienes. Isoflavones and omega-3 fatty acids also inhibit inflammation. These substances also serve as mild forms of estrogens, and thus protect against the more severe estrogens that promote cancer.

Whole or ground-up and roasted flaxseeds have been shown to reduce the risk of prostate swelling and prostate cancer in men. This is in contrast with the research done on flaxseed oil, which may have a pro-inflammatory effect on the prostate. Recent studies suggest that flaxseed oil may increase the risk of prostate cancer. My advice: Eat the seeds, not the oil.

Flaxseeds are tiny. When roasted and ground up, they become small, crunchy particles that can serve as a condiment on beans and vegetables and, in Phase 2, on grains and noodles. Flaxseeds have a mild, nutty flavor that doesn't intrude on the taste of the foods they are used to enhance.

Pumpkin seeds also contain bioflavonoids, isoflavones, and omega-3 fatty acids, though not in the quantities possessed by flaxseeds. Use pumpkin seeds as a condiment on vegetables and beans, too. Two points of caution: Pumpkin seeds, while rich in omega-3s, do contain higher levels of fat than flaxseeds and therefore should be used sparingly, especially during Phase 1. Second, many people find that pumpkin seeds cause some mild stomach distress, especially when consumed alone as a snack. During Phase 1, use pumpkin seeds only as a condiment on your vegetables or beans. They are very pleasing, with a crunchy, mild flavor. During Phase 2, add pumpkin seeds to your brown rice and other grains. They make a delicious condiment on grains and add another anti-inflammatory food to your diet.

Fruit

Studies have consistently shown that people who eat high quantities of vegetables and fruits have lower rates of heart disease, stroke, high blood pressure, diabetes, and all forms of cancer than those who don't. In fact, a diet rich in fruits and vegetables protects against all degenerative diseases. Health authorities have been recommending for more than a decade that we eat at least five servings of fruits and vegetables per day. We have already seen many reasons why we should eat vegetables. Though fruit is less abundant in its vitamin, mineral, antioxidant, and phytochemical content, it is nonetheless a rich source of many important plant chemicals, including antioxidants and flavonoids. Fruit also contains plenty of fiber, much of which is soluble fiber that reduces the cholesterol content of your blood. Taken together, these traits reduce inflammation, control blood sugar, insulin levels, boost your immune system, and inhibit many of the factors that create serious illness.

Avoid dried fruit because of its high simple-sugar content. Without the water content, dried fruit becomes a very concentrated source of calories. Whole, fresh fruit is rich in nutrients, fiber, and water, which means it will fill you up before loading you down with calories.

In the Phase 1 regimen, I recommend that you consume at least 13 servings of fruit per day. The many fruits available to us include apples, apricots, bananas, blueberries, blackberries, cherries, cantaloupe and other melons, grapes, Kiwi fruit, nectarines, oranges, grapefruits, lemons, plums, raisins, strawberries, tangerines, and raspberries.

Condiments, Sauces, and Spices

Use salad dressings that are fat-free and low in calories. Avoid salt intake, especially if you are salt-sensitive and have high blood pressure. Here are some dressings, condiments, and sauces that can be used in the Phase 1 program.

* Balsamic vinegar
* Brown-rice vinegar
* Wine vinegars
* Fresh, grated ginger root
* Horseradish
* Lemon juice
* Mustard
* Pepper
* Sauerkraut (low-sodium if you are salt-sensitive and have high blood pressure)
* Salsa
* Salt substitute
* Miso (use in soup and sauces only if you are not hypertensive and not salt-sensitive)
* Garlic, onions, and scallions

Exercise: Take a Walk and Save Your Life

The only exercise I recommend during Phase 1 is walking. Walk three to seven days a week, depending on your current state of health. Do so at a leisurely pace. Do not power-walk.

Before you begin your walking regimen, I urge you to see your doctor and undergo a full medical checkup. Tell your doctor that you would like to begin walking daily and ask if there are any restrictions on how much you should walk, or how far. Follow your doctor's recommendations.

Start out your program by walking for 30 minutes a day at a comfortable pace. Distance and speed do not matter as much as time. Stroll if you like. In fact, if you have been told by your doctor that you have heart disease, or if you have had a heart attack, I encourage you to stroll, at least during the first few weeks of your program.

Meanwhile, remain faithful to your Phase 1 program. This will bring down blood cholesterol, C-reactive protein, homocysteine, fibrinogen, and other important blood values, all of which means that the chances of having a heart attack are dropping precipitously. As your health improves, increase the number of times you walk per week. With continued improvement, increase the distance you walk.

As for speed, walk at a pace that will allow you to carry on a conversation without feeling out of breath or straining for breath. If you are struggling to breathe as you walk, stop immediately. Rest until you have fully recovered your breath, and then return home. If you resume walking, do so at a slower pace. Do not overexert yourself.

As your health improves, you will witness a significant improvement in your fitness and stamina. Let your body guide you as you increase distance and speed. Do not push yourself. As long as you are walking and eating well, your health and fitness will naturally improve. Allow your body to recover at its natural pace.

Experience Improvement in Seven Days

As your cholesterol level falls, the cholesterol inside the cholesterol plaques begins to drain out. Inflammation starts to cool as well. Both of these improvements make the plaques far less volatile and unstable, and less likely to rupture and cause a heart attack. The draining of the cholesterol pools is the first step in reversing the creation of atherosclerotic plaques.

On the Phase 1 program it takes about seven days to begin the process of lowering your blood cholesterol resulting from the consumption of dietary saturated fat and excess calories. This means your liver will have to draw on your body stores of fat and cholesterol, including those in the plaques of your arteries, to obtain the necessary materials to make more cholesterol, thereby beginning the process of draining the plaques and moving you away from the risk of having a heart attack or stroke. This is why I urge those who are in immediate danger of having a heart attack to adopt and adhere to Phase 1 until all the goals described above are reached.

Phase 1a: An Intermediate Step

I usually do not switch my patients immediately from Phase 1 to Phase 2. Instead, I encourage people to adopt an intermediate step by including in their Phase 1 diet two whole-grain dishes per day. I call this intermediate step Phase 1a. The diagram below shows the Phase 1a pyramid.

The breakdown of the foods is as follows:

- 17 servings of vegetables
- 10 servings of fruits
- 2 servings of whole grains and cereals

Phase 1a is a transition to a wider diet and an overall long-term healthy way of eating. It also gives you the opportunity to start learning how to prepare whole grains to make them delicious and rewarding, before you take on the entire Phase 2 program. I do this partly to allow you the time to get accustomed to grain as a primary dish. In fact, for most cultures around the

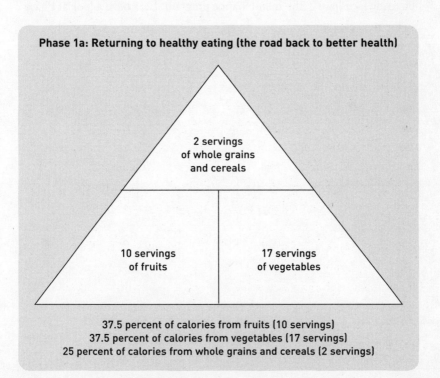

Phase 1a: Returning to healthy eating (the road back to better health)

2 servings
of whole grains
and cereals

10 servings
of fruits

17 servings
of vegetables

37.5 percent of calories from fruits (10 servings)
37.5 percent of calories from vegetables (17 servings)
25 percent of calories from whole grains and cereals (2 servings)

world, whole grain is the central staple food, much as meat and animal foods are for Americans.

I recommend that you follow Phase 1a for up to a month before adopting Phase 2.

When you've learned to prepare whole grains, you'll wonder how you ever lived without them. Whole grains are delicious, high-energy foods. They're rich in complex carbohydrates, which are slow-burning fuel that provides long-lasting energy. They are also great sources of nutrition, including vitamin E, B vitamins, minerals, and protein. Grain, as you know, is a wonderful source of fiber, including soluble fibers, which lower cholesterol. They vary in flavors and cooking times. Occasionally combine grains with beans to make delicious and satisfying dishes. People who eat grain regularly often say that it makes them feel less anxious, more emotionally centered and grounded.

There is a wide variety of whole grains, as you will learn in the section on whole grains in chapter 10.

Once you are out of danger and have achieved the Phase 1 goals, you will be ready for Phase 2, the maintenance program. Let's have a look at Phase 2 in the next chapter.

10

Phase 2 of the Fleming STOP INFLAMMATION NOW! Program

PHASE 2 OF THE FLEMING STOP INFLAM-
MATION NOW! Program is designed to maintain the achievements you have
made in Phase 1. Phase 2 gives you lots of freedom, even as it sustains all the
benefits that you have achieved with Phase 1. Phase 2 will allow you to have
greater latitude in restaurants and when you travel. You will be able to go to
seafood, Italian, natural-foods, Chinese, and Japanese restaurants, just to
name a few, and order foods that fall well within the Phase 2 guidelines.

Whenever you dine out, please do adhere to the following guidelines.

1. Request of your server that food be prepared without oil; if that isn't possible, use only olive oil, and only sparingly.
2. Make sure your meals include lots of vegetables.
3. Request that none of your vegetables be cooked in butter or margarine.
   Ask that they be steamed or lightly sautéed in olive oil. Be sure to remain
   within the Phase 2 guidelines for olive oil.

4. Request that any animal foods that you order be limited to 3.5 ounces, or the size of a deck of cards.
5. Avoid extra cheeses or heavy creams or sauces containing these foods. They're loaded with calories and will cause rapid weight gain.
6. Eat salad with low-fat dressing. Bring your own dressing if your favorite restaurants don't provide them.

Phase 2: An Overview of the More Varied Diet

Phase 2 is much more varied than Phase 1, including vegetables, fruits, whole grains, pasta, and small amounts of animal foods. The proportions of these foods are shown in the Phase 2 pyramid below.

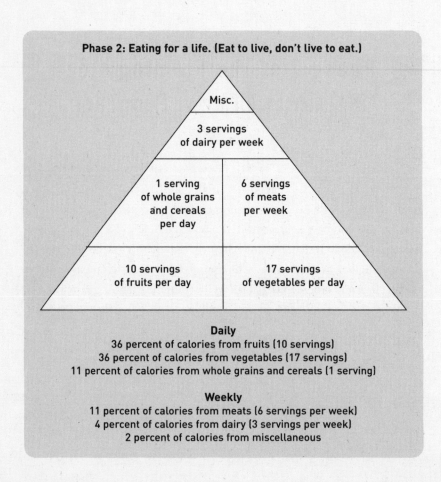

Phase 2: Eating for a life. (Eat to live, don't live to eat.)

Misc.

3 servings
of dairy per week

1 serving
of whole grains
and cereals
per day

6 servings
of meats
per week

10 servings
of fruits per day

17 servings
of vegetables per day

Daily
36 percent of calories from fruits (10 servings)
36 percent of calories from vegetables (17 servings)
11 percent of calories from whole grains and cereals (1 serving)

Weekly
11 percent of calories from meats (6 servings per week)
4 percent of calories from dairy (3 servings per week)
2 percent of calories from miscellaneous

The Phase 2 maintenance diet comprises 15 percent protein, 70 percent complex carbohydrates, and 15 percent fat. The ratio of polyunsaturated and monounsaturated fats to saturated is 2:1. Saturated fat intake is restricted to 5 grams or less per day. This is easily accomplished by limiting your intake of animal foods to 3.5 ounces of fish, red meat, eggs, or chicken.

Phase 2 Foods

On the Phase 2 diet you can eat the following foods:

- *All the vegetables listed in Phase 1.* These include all the green and leafy vegetables; all the white, yellow, orange, and red varieties; all the tubers; all the roots; legumes and legume products; and sea vegetables.
- *All the fruits listed in Phase 1.*
- *Whole grains.* Whole grains such as brown rice, barley, and millet are abundant sources of complex carbohydrates, which provide long-lasting energy without weight gain. People whose diets are based on whole grains and vegetables are typically lean and have no trouble maintaining their ideal body weight. Whole grains are rich in fiber, nutrients, and antioxidants, including vitamin E.
- *Noodles and pasta.* There is an incredible variety of noodles and pastas made from a wide array of grains and vegetables. Contrary to widely held belief, noodles and pastas are not particularly fattening. It's what you put on the noodles that increases your weight. If you combine pasta with vegetables to make pasta primavera, you will be eating a moderate- to low-calorie food. And you'll be getting complex carbohydrates and lots of nutrition.
- *Animal foods.* During Phase 2 you may eat small portions of fish, skinless poultry, eggs, and lean meats. Six servings of flesh foods, such as fish, skinless chicken, or lean meat, are permitted each week. Animal foods are limited to a 3.5-ounce serving (about the size of a deck of cards). Eggs are limited to two per week.
- *Skim milk and low-fat dairy products.* Three servings of dairy products, including skim milk and low-fat cheese, are permitted each week.
- *Nuts and seeds.* Roasted and ground-up flaxseeds and pumpkin seeds are allowed as recommended for Phase 1. About a half cup each of walnuts and almonds per week is permitted in Phase 2.

- *Vegetable oils.* The preferred oils are olive, sesame, and safflower. These oils are low in saturated fat and high in mono- and polyunsaturated fats. Oil is liquid fat. All fats are limited to about a tablespoon a day.
- A *daily supplement.* Same as that recommended for Phase 1.
- *Beverages.* Same as those recommended for Phase 1.

Use Phase 2 to provide ongoing support and enhancement of your heart and overall health. The addition of whole grains and animal foods will very likely give you greater strength and increased endurance. Grains are energy foods. Small amounts of animal products can also increase your sense of strength, vitality, and personal power. However, do not overdo them. Any increase in animal foods can elevate inflammation and have serious consequences for your health.

Phase 2: In Depth

One of the keys to Phase 2 is to limit the total calorie intake to about 1,500 calories a day, or 10 calories per pound of ideal body weight. So if your ideal body weight is 130 pounds, you would consume 1,300 calories per day; if it's 170 pounds, you would consume 1,700 calories per day.

Promote Weight Loss on Phase 2

One of the ways to ensure that you sustain all the health goals that you achieved on Phase 1 is to make sure that you do not gain weight on Phase 2.

To enjoy the more varied Phase 2 program and still lose weight, do the following:

- Make vegetables and fruits the center of your diet.
- Limit total fat intake to 15 percent of calories; one of the ways to do this is by eating only small portions (3.5 ounces) of animal foods per day.
- Eat one or two small servings (one cup or less) of cooked whole grain daily, such as amaranth, barley, brown rice, buckwheat, millet, or quinoa.
- Avoid overly refined breads and other baked flour products, including whole-wheat bread. Grain products should be loaded with fiber, and refined grains, which don't have much fiber, are missing much of their nutritional value.

- Avoid sugar and processed foods.
- Eat low-fat animal products, such as fish, the white meat of chicken, or lean beef. Limit the serving size to 3.5 ounces, or about the size of a deck of cards. The dark meat of chicken and the skin both have more calories than the white meat.
- Use only olive, sesame, and safflower oils and limit consumption of oil to one tablespoon a day.
- Use low-fat salad dressings, sauces, and condiments (see chapter 14).
- As in Phase 1, do not eat after 7 P.M. All food consumed after 7 P.M. is converted to triglycerides and body fat.
- Phase 2 allows dairy products for those who want to drink small amounts of milk or eat small quantities of cheese. In order to sustain optimal weight, drink only skim milk and eat only skim-milk cheeses. Limit milk products to three servings per week.
- Phase 2 allows small amounts of pasta and noodles to be eaten. In order to ensure that you don't get too many calories, eat pasta without oil and cook your noodles with vegetables to make pasta primavera. The veggies will add nutients, flavor, and fiber to the meal, without adding calories. The pasta will be delicious and satisfying—and all on a low-calorie meal.

Keep in mind that pasta is not a high-calorie food. Three and a half ounces of pasta with tomato sauce and cooked vegetables provides about 160 calories. That's less than the same-size serving of chicken and about 60 calories less than a 3.5-ounce serving of sirloin steak. Pasta is also rich in complex carbs; it provides a significant amount of protein—one cup of cooked spaghetti provides almost as much protein as a whole egg. Pasta also provides B vitamins, iron, and fiber. As long as you don't add cheese or oil, noodles contain virtually no fat. It's the Parmesan cheese and olive oil that give pasta a bad name.

Whole Grains

The following is a list of the whole grains that I recommend you eat regularly as part of the Phase 2 program.

AMARANTH

A tiny grain that was cultivated by the Native-American Aztecs, amaranth is one of the most nutritionally abundant grains available. It's rich in protein, calcium, folic acid, magnesium, and iron. Amaranth can be boiled in 30 minutes. Cook with vegetables or alone.

BARLEY

Barley contains folic acid, magnesium, phosphorus, potassium, and zinc. It's also a good source of cholesterol-lowering soluble fiber. This versatile grain comes in whole form or cracked, which is often referred to as "pearled." Even when pearled, barley's core is still intact. Whole barley takes about 55 minutes to cook, whereas the pearled variety can be prepared in about 30 minutes. Add a pinch of salt to the water to help the grain open and make it to soften more rapidly. Barley is delicious and hearty in soups and stews. It's wonderful when prepared with hearty vegetables, such as carrots, onions, leeks, and the exotic shiitake mushrooms.

BROWN RICE

Like barley, corn, and oats, brown rice is a rich source of soluble fiber, which means it can lower blood cholesterol. Brown rice provides an abundant supply of complex carbohydrates for energy. It is rich in vitamin E and also contains B vitamins such as thiamine and niacin, iron, phosphorus, and magnesium. Brown rice is a good source of protein as well, because it contains the amino acid lysine, which is often missing from grains. Three varieties of brown rice—short grain, medium length, and long grain—are grown. The short-grain brown rice is heartier and richer; the long-grain is lighter and more appropriate for summer and warmer climes.

Short-grain rice takes longer to cook than long-grain, and can be boiled or pressure-cooked in about 45 minutes; long-grain can be boiled in about 30 minutes.

To pressure-cook brown rice, place in the cooker approximately two cups of water for every cup of rice. Add a pinch of salt to the water and grain to allow the grain to open and cook more rapidly. Fasten the lid to the pressure cooker and set on a high flame. Allow the pot to come to pressure (it usually takes about 10 minutes). Once the regulator whistles, turn the flame to low and allow to simmer for 40 to 45 minutes.

BUCKWHEAT

Buckwheat is actually a grass rather than a true grain, but has served as a grain substitute for many cold-weather climates, such as Russia and Lithuania, where it is known as kasha. Buckwheat is quick-cooking—it can be prepared in 15 minutes—and has a delicious, nutty flavor. It can be cooked with carrots, sauerkraut, and other vegetables.

MILLET

Don't be fooled by millet's tiny size: it's a nutritional goldmine. Loaded with thiamine and other B vitamins, millet also contains significant amounts of magnesium, copper, iron, potassium, and protein. Millet is wonderful when cooked with other vegetables, such as carrots. When cooked with cauliflower, it combines to make a delicious, mashed potato–like consistency. Millet is especially good when cooked in a soup stock. Millet takes only 25 minutes to prepare, but add plenty of water: 1.5 cups of water to 1 cup of millet.

OATS

Oats provide remarkably high levels of protein, iron, manganese, copper, folic acid, vitamin E, and zinc. Oats can be purchased in several forms, including rolled, instant rolled, steel-cut, and whole. Rolled oats take about 5 to 6 minutes to cook. Steel-cut oats are more nutritious than rolled. They are also more crunchy and flavorful. They need to be boiled for about 20 minutes. Whole oats are the most time-consuming and are often impractical. If you like whole oats, put them in a slow-cooker and cook them overnight, or soak them overnight and then boil for 5 to 7 minutes. Oats make for a delicious breakfast cereal, especially when cooked with raisins. After cooking, add roasted ground-up flaxseeds, wheat germ, and a sweetener, such as maple or rice syrup or barley malt.

QUINOA

Pronounced "keen-WAH," quinoa is often referred to as a supergrain for its rich supply of protein, potassium, riboflavin, magnesium, zinc, copper, manganese, and folic acid. Quinoa is also a quick-cooking grain. Combine a half cup of grain and a cup of water and boil for 15 minutes. Voilà! You've got a cup of delicious, fluffy quinoa.

WHEAT

Wheat is especially nutritious. It contains high levels of protein, vitamin E, iron, B vitamins, magnesium, and manganese.

Most of us only know wheat as a flour used for wheat bread, but wheat comes in many forms.

Wheat berries that have not been cracked are very flavorful, hearty, and chewy. Soak them overnight and boil for about 70 minutes. Combine with vegetables such as carrots and onions to produce a delicious whole-grain meal.

Bulgur (cracked wheat) is known to most people as the basis for a salad called tabouli, made with olive oil, lemon juice, chopped tomatoes, and parsley. Boxed mixes are widely available and easy to prepare.

Couscous is a small, white grain that's made from semolina and contains some B vitamins and iron. Couscous requires less than 30 minutes to prepare. It's usually cooked with a medley of vegetables, such as peas, carrots, and corn.

Farina is a more refined version of bulgur that's cooked as an old-fashioned hot breakfast cereal.

Wheat germ, a wonderful topping for breakfast cereals, is a great source of vitamin E, thiamine, riboflavin, and protein. Keep it refrigerated.

The Japanese produce a variety of interesting and delicious wheat-derived products, including fu, a delicious puffed-wheat gluten product that's chewy and rich in protein and is used in soups and stews; and seitan, a meat-substitute that is extremely rich in protein. Like fu, seitan (pronounced "say-tan") is delicious in stews, soups, stews, noodle dishes, and vegetable medleys.

Many people are sensitive to the gluten in wheat and experience allergic symptoms and indigestion whenever they eat wheat products. If you suffer from any type of chronic sinus congestion, runny nose, unexplained indigestion, bloatedness, constipation, or diarrhea, stop eating wheat products and any food containing wheat gluten. The elimination of wheat and gluten may bring about a cessation of your symptoms.

Emphasize Anti-inflammatory Vegetables and Fruits

Remember that you are eating to be healthy and happy, which means that you want to eat lots of anti-inflammatory foods on Phase 2. Highlight the following foods in your diet:

- Cruciferous vegetables, including broccoli, cauliflower, collard greens, kale, and mustard greens.
- Allium vegetables, including garlic, onions, scallions, and leeks.
- Blueberries, grapes, plums, and other anti-inflammatory fruits.
- Vitamin C–rich foods, including broccoli, leafy green vegetables, and citrus fruits.
- Flaxseeds (seeds are limited to one teaspoon per day on Phase 1).
- Omega-3 polyunsaturated fats (found in cold-water fish for Phase 2).
- Walnuts, almonds, and pumpkin seeds. These foods inhibit blood-clot formation and are anti-inflammatory. They also inhibit tumor formation.
- Fiber-rich foods, which bind with hormones and the inflammatory prostaglandins.

Low-Fat Fish

In Phase 2, fish is a good source of omega-3 fatty acids.

Bluefish—an especially high source of omega-3 fatty acids
Cod
Flounder—cold-water ocean fish, rich in omega-3 fatty acids
Haddock—cold-water ocean fish, rich in omega-3 fatty acids
Halibut—cold-water ocean fish, rich in omega-3 fatty acids
Herring—especially abundant in omega-3 fatty acids
Mackerel—especially rich in omega-3 fatty acids
Mahi mahi
Orange roughy
Pollock
Pompano
Red snapper
Sablefish—especially rich in omega-3 fatty acids
Salmon—especially rich in omega-3 fatty acids
Sardines—especially rich in omega-3 fatty acids
Sole
Swordfish
Tuna—especially rich in omega-3 fatty acids
Whitefish

Other Animal Foods

The white meat of poultry, cooked and eaten without the skin, is lower in calories and saturated fat than red meats (i.e., beef and lamb) or pork.

Nuts and Seeds

Phase 2 permits small amounts of walnuts and almonds, along with flax- and pumpkin seeds, which are described in Phase 1 (see chapter 9). The fat in walnuts and almonds is primarily polyunsaturated, which means that they lower blood cholesterol, and monounsaturated fats, which do not change cholesterol levels. However, both nuts have been shown to lower overall cholesterol, including LDL levels. Walnuts contain the antioxidant selenium. Researchers have found that people who eat nuts tend to be more satisfied by their diets than those who do not eat nuts. Nut eaters tend to be leaner and healthier than their non-nut-eating counterparts. Still, I recommend that people limit their intake, because nuts contain significant amounts of calories. Eat only a half cup of each per week.

Tea

I urge my patients to abstain from all beverages that contain caffeine, but if you must consume caffeine, the only beverages that I would recommend are black and green tea, both of which contain significant amounts of bioflavonoids and antioxidants, substances that reduce inflammation and boost immune function. Scientists at Tufts University have found that one cup of black or green tea has greater antioxidant powers than half a cup of broccoli, carrots, spinach, or strawberries.

Studies have found that tea drinkers have lower incidences of cancers of the esophagus, kidneys, bladder, and colon than non-tea drinkers. Animal studies have shown that tea inhibits cancer cells from forming.

Tea has significant anti-inflammatory effects as well. Dutch researchers have found that people who drink tea daily have half the risk of suffering a fatal heart attack as non-tea drinkers.

This research is still in its early stages, but the findings are consistent and persuasive. Tea appears to boost immune function, help fight cancer, and prevent heart disease. That's a lot in a little cup. So drop the coffee and have a cup of tea. You'll relax more and maybe enjoy just a little more peace of mind.

The Risks of
High-Protein Diets

*

THE EPIDEMIC OF OVERWEIGHT IS DRIV-
ing tens of millions of people to extreme and dangerous behaviors. It's easy
to understand why: Millions of people are gaining weight, even as they try to
lose it. That kind of frustration leads to all kinds of imbalanced and unhealthy
decisions, not the least of which is to adopt a high-protein diet.

High-protein diets are now the fashion. Remarkably, they are even being
recommended to people by some medical doctors. One cardiologist told me
that he knows that high-protein diets cause significant health problems, yet
he still recommends them to some of his patients. I could hardly believe
what I was hearing. Why? I asked him. Because overweight is worse than the
problems associated with high-protein diets, he said. That statement is de-
batable, in part because high-protein diets will not solve our epidemic of
overweight, as most people who have tried them already know. In any case,
according to this man's twisted logic, you cannot have both weight loss and
good health at the same time. You have to choose one or the other. That kind

of reasoning (or the lack of it) is symptomatic of just how confused and lost we are today in matters of health and weight.

The fact is that high-protein diets elevate most of the risk factors for heart disease. Those risk factors injure the heart and result in coronary heart disease. High-protein diets also cause calcium loss and weakening of bones; if sustained, this can lead to osteoporosis. These regimens, which are based largely on animal foods, are deficient in fiber, antioxidants, vitamins, minerals, and phytochemicals. Thus, they often result in constipation, digestive problems, and immune weakness. High-protein diets are high-fat diets. The U.S. surgeon general has concluded, based on much scientific evidence, that high-fat diets increase your risk of cancer, including cancers of the breast, colon, and prostate. Finally, studies show that high-protein diets can cause significant kidney damage and can create kidney stones.

The irony is that most people cannot adhere to high-protein diets for very long, which means that they injure their health and usually regain the weight they lost. How's that for frustrating?!

For many years, I have been treating people who come to me with heart disease and weight problems. A great many of my patients were on high-protein diets before seeing me. How did you feel on that diet? I ask them. Terrible, they tell me. They are usually constipated and uncomfortable in their bodies. Many suffered from digestive disorders, joint pain, reduced energy, poor sleep, and food cravings, especially cravings for carbohydrate-rich foods. Eventually, those cravings became so strong that they overcame the person's willpower and sent him or her off on a processed-food binge, which usually resulted in even greater weight gain.

Nevertheless, more and more people today are adopting high-fat diets, thanks to an array of promises made by their proponents. Among the most enticing of these promises is that you can eat high-fat foods, lose weight, and experience improved health.

Those who have been on these diets know from experience that that cannot happen. Others know intuitively that you cannot be on a diet of steak, bacon, eggs, sausage, heavy cream, ice cream, and cheese and expect to be healthy. Unfortunately, until a short time ago, there was little or no research to support or refute these claims. I changed all of that with two studies on the effects of high-protein diets on health, and especially on cardiovascular risk factors. Both my studies showed that people who follow these diets for longer than three months experience significant elevation in cardiovascular risk factors. One of the studies showed a clear reduction of blood flow to the heart in those who followed a high-protein diet for one year.

It's true that up until that three-month point, people do lose weight and experience a drop in cholesterol and triglycerides, as reported recently by Duke University researchers. However, from three to six months later, health starts to take a decided turn for the worse.

Allow me to explain my two studies, starting with the most recent (Fleming 2002).

I randomly assigned 100 volunteers to four groups and placed each group on a separate diet. I then followed the effects of these diets on each subject's blood values over the course of one year. The four diets were as follows:

Diet 1. The Fleming Phase 1 diet, composed of vegetables and fruits. I referred to it in the study as the 10 percent fat diet, meaning that it derived only 10 percent of its total calories from fat. On this diet, people were allowed to eat as much food as they wanted, as long as they ate food permitted on the Phase 1 diet. Even so, their total calorie intake amounted to 1,300 to 1,400 calories per day.

Diet 2. The Fleming Phase 2 diet, composed of whole grains, vegetables, and fruit. This diet derived 15 percent of its total calories from fat. It restricted calories to 1,500 to 1,600 calories per day.

Diet 3. The diet was essentially the one recommended by the American Heart Association, which was composed of 20 to 30 percent total calories in fat. This regimen did not restrict calories. People ate diets that contained between 2,000 and 2,200 calories per day.

Diet 4. High-protein, high-fat, low-carbohydrate. This diet derived 55 to 65 percent of its total calories from fat. Ten percent of its calories came from carbohydrates. The number of calories consumed each day was between 1,400 and 1,500.

In addition to following their respective diets, all the study participants were encouraged to follow the same exercise regime, which was to stretch for 15 minutes and walk for 30 minutes, three to five times per week.

The Results: New Insights into
Those Inflated Promises

Five very important findings jumped out from the study immediately.

1. You can lose weight and dramatically improve your health. The people who followed Diet 1, composed of vegetables and fruits, lost significant amounts of weight (18 percent of their total body weight, on average) and saw all their risk factors for heart disease fall into the healthy ranges. In fact, the vegetable-and-fruit diet was far more effective as a weight-loss diet than the high-protein diet. People who followed Diet 2, composed of whole grains, vegetables, and fruit, also lost weight and saw their cardio-vascular risk factors fall.

2. There is no magic weight-loss principle for the high-protein diets. Every-one in my study lost weight, no matter what diet they were on, as long as they ate fewer calories than were needed to sustain their current weight. That means that the age-old principle for weight loss is still the principle that matters most: If you eat fewer calories than you need to sustain your current weight, you will lose weight. It doesn't matter what diet you choose. The same rule applies.

3. The third lesson was this: During the first 12 weeks, or three months, everyone experienced a reduction in their risk factors, including total cholesterol, LDL cholesterol, triglycerides, C-reactive protein, homocys-teine, fibrinogen, and lipoprotein (a). This occurred because there was a reduction in calorie consumption. Fewer calories means less stress on the liver. When the liver is not dealing with the overabundance of calories, it starts to cleanse itself by removing toxic substances that long have been stored in its tissues. The simple truth is that the human body functions better on a calorie-reduced diet.

   However, after three months, the overall fat content, especially satu-rated fat, consumed on the high-protein diet began to take its toll. At that point, all the risk factors for those on the high-protein regimen began to climb. By the end of one year, the people on the high-protein program ex-perienced a significant increase in virtually all of their major risk factors for heart disease. Why did this occur? Because it takes the liver about three months to adapt to its new conditions. Once it adapted to the lower calories in the high-protein diet, it was forced to deal with the relatively high proportions of fat and protein, both of which placed a new toxic burden on the organ. The saturated fat and protein placed a new toxic burden on the liver, which in turn made all the cardiovascular risk factors go up.

4. The fourth lesson learned was that everyone adhered to their respective diets for one year. I believe that this was due to consistent monitoring by my staff and me. People will stick to their diets if they are coached by their physicians and their doctor's staff. I followed these people very closely. Study participants came into my office every six weeks to have their blood tests performed, to get answers to their questions, and to receive encouragement to remain on the program. This type of consistent follow-up gave people a strong incentive to stick to their diets. Left on their own, people would not have complied with the diets as well as they did, I believe. All of which illustrates for me that doctors must be involved in their patients' efforts to change their eating habits.

5. And finally, my study was yet another reminder that the American Heart Association diet is not a weight-loss diet. The people who followed the 20 to 30 percent fat diet gained little benefit against disease and on average lost little weight. This is especially disappointing because many people still view the American Heart Association as a scientific organization dedicated to good health. Which means that anyone who adopts the AHA regimen, adheres to it to the letter, and expects it to reduce his or her risk factors may be disappointed. This is one of the reasons laypeople have such grave doubts about science and scientists today. Many follow the advice and fail to get the results they had hoped for, or were promised.

All of which also calls into question any study that compares the AHA diet with a high-protein diet, which is what the Duke University study did. What's the point? Any comparison between the two is bound to make the high-protein diet look good—at least when it comes to weight loss. This is one of the reasons why proponents of the high-protein diet were celebrating after Duke researchers released their preliminary results. "Look at this," people said. "The high-protein diet caused weight loss and a drop in triglycerides and cholesterol! And it was better than the American Heart Association diet. Isn't that the diet that cardiologists are recommending?! They don't know what they're talking about."

Like many people, I was surprised by the AHA's response, so sure was I that they would point out the flaws in the study. Surely, I thought, they would point out that the reason for the greater weight loss on the high-protein diet was the result of fewer calories being eaten. Surely, I thought, they wouldn't let this stand. So I called the AHA and, while the response was unexpected, it was right. The AHA doesn't have a diet! There is nothing in their literature that says reduce the number of calories you eat. The recommendation is to avoid exceeding a certain percentage of your calories in fat or to cut down the amount of cholesterol you eat in any given day—depending on the type of diet. It isn't designed to reduce your weight. So I concede, the Duke study had clearly shown that if you cut calories you lose weight. (For those of you interested in physics, the second law of thermodynamics still applies!)

Let's have a closer look at the findings.

Weight Loss: Vegetables and Fruit Win—by a Mile

The diet that led to the greatest weight loss was Diet 1, which is Phase 1 of the Fleming Program. Diets 2 and 4, the whole grain-vegetables-and-fruit diet, and the high-protein diet, respectively, were just about equal in creating weight loss. Diet 3, the AHA-similar diet, was the least effective at creating weight loss. The weight loss after one year for each diet was as follows:

Diet 1. People who followed Diet 1 lost 18 percent—nearly one fifth—of their body weight. A person who weighed 200 pounds and was significantly overweight lost about 40 pounds in one year. A person who weighed 300 pounds lost about 60 pounds after one year. Keep in mind that these examples are based on average weight loss. Some people lost much more; others lost less.

Diet 2. People who followed Diet 2 lost on average 12 percent of their body weight. Those who weighed 200 pounds and were overweight lost on average 24 pounds. Those who weighed 300 pounds lost on average 36 pounds.

Diet 3. On average, the people who followed the AHA-similar diet did not lose weight. The only people who lost weight on Diet 3 were those who weighed more than 200 pounds before the study began and ate a diet that contained 2,000 calories per day. That diet would bring them down to 200 pounds, approximately. (Remember, you need 10 calories per pound to sustain your current weight. A 200-pound person will remain at 200 pounds if he or she eats 2,000 calories per day.)

Diet 4. Those who followed the high-protein, high-fat, low-carbohydrate diet lost on average 13 percent of their body weight. That means that if they weighed 200 pounds and were overweight, they lost on average about 26 pounds. A 300-pound person could lose 39 pounds.

Contrary to widespread belief, the high-protein diet was not the most effective weight-loss program. The vegetable-and-fruit diet was far more effective at producing weight loss. It was also the greatest promoter of good health.

Good Health and Weight Loss Can Be Achieved

My study was designed to discover what the effects of each diet were over a year-long period. In addition to weight, I monitored eight other major risk factors for heart disease in each of the study participants:

- Total cholesterol
- LDL cholesterol
- HDL cholesterol
- The total cholesterol-to-HDL ratio
- Triglycerides
- Homocysteine
- Lipoprotein (a)
- Fibrinogen

Let's look at how each of these risk factors were affected after one year on each of the four diets.

TOTAL CHOLESTEROL

Diet 1. The people on Diet 1, vegetables and fruit, experienced a 39.1 percent drop in total cholesterol. A person who had a cholesterol level of 200 mg/dL would see a reduction of nearly 80 mg, to about 120 mg/dL.

Diet 2. The people on Diet 2—whole grains, vegetables, and fruit—experienced a 30.4 percent drop in total cholesterol.

Diet 3. Those on the AHA-like moderate-fat diet, with a total fat content of 20 to 30 percent, experienced a 5 percent drop in total cholesterol.

Diet 4. The people on the high-protein, high-fat diet experienced an increase in total cholesterol of 4.3 percent.

LDL CHOLESTEROL: THE DISEASE-CAUSING CHOLESTEROL

Diet 1. The participants who followed Diet 1 experienced a 52 percent decline in LDL cholesterol in 12 months. LDL was essentially cut in half. That means that inflammation dropped significantly, and the people on Diet 1 very likely experienced reversal of cholesterol plaques, or atherosclerosis.

Diet 2. Participants on Diet 2 experienced a 38.8 percent drop in LDL cholesterol, also a significant reduction that very likely resulted in reversal of atherosclerosis.

Diet 3. Those who followed the AHA-like moderate-fat diet experienced a 6.1 percent drop in LDL—not a particularly significant reduction and unlikely to affect coronary artery disease to any significant extent.

Diet 4. Those on the high-protein, high-fat diet saw their LDL levels go up 6 percent. In other words, the risk of heart disease, heart attack, and stroke was now increasing.

HDL CHOLESTEROL: THE GOOD CHOLESTEROL

Diet 1. Those following Diet 1 experienced a 9 percent increase in HDL cholesterol, which translates into greater protection against heart attack and stroke.

Diet 2. Those on Diet 2 experienced a 3.6 percent increase in HDL, also a significant improvement.

Diet 3. Those on the AHA-similar diet had decreases in their HDL of 1.5 percent, never a good sign.

Diet 4. Those on the high-protein, high-fat diet experienced a decrease in HDL of 5.8 percent, a significant drop in good cholesterol. Again, an indication that liver function was declining.

RATIO OF TOTAL CHOLESTEROL TO HDL CHOLESTEROL

As you know, cardiologists prefer to see total cholesterol-to-HDL ratios of 4:1 or lower, say, 3:1. In this case, a lower ratio is viewed as an improvement in heart health, because it means that the HDL cholesterol is increasing, relative to the total cholesterol. That's what every cardiologist wants to see.

Diet 1. People on Diet 1 experienced a 45.8 percent reduction in the ratio of total cholesterol to HDL. A remarkable improvement in heart health.

Diet 2. People on Diet 2 experienced a 34.7 percent reduction in the ratio of total cholesterol to HDL. Another dramatic reduction in risk.

Diet 3. Those on the AHA-like diet experienced a 5.3 percent drop in the ratio.

Diet 4. Those on the high-protein, high-fat diet experienced a 9.8 percent increase in the ratio of total cholesterol to HDL. That means that those on the high protein, high-fat diet saw their risk of heart attack and stroke go up.

TRIGLYCERIDES: BLOOD FATS THAT TURN INTO BLOOD CHOLESTEROL

Diet 1. Those on Diet 1 experienced a 37.3 percent drop in triglycerides. Thus, a major risk factor for heart disease was reduced by more than a third.

Diet 2. Those on Diet 2 had virtually the same result: 36.9 percent decline in triglycerides.

Diet 3. People on the AHA-similar diet experienced an increase in triglycerides of 1 percent. Admittedly, that's only a small increase, but if you are on a diet, you expect to get better. That increase in blood fats was probably the result of the high-calorie content of this diet.

Diet 4. People on the high-protein, high-fat diet experienced an interesting roller-coaster ride with regard to triglycerides. During the first four months, triglycerides fell 3.5 percent. By the eighth month, however, triglycerides were up 3.3 percent, and by 12 months, they had increased 5.5 percent. One of the reasons triglycerides go up, of course, is consumption of fat, particularly saturated fat.

HOMOCYSTEINE: THE AMINO ACID THAT INJURES YOUR ARTERIES

Diet 1. On Diet 1, homocysteine levels were reduced by 13.6 percent. That means that there were fewer injuries to the arteries and less oxidation. Any plaques that did exist were far less volatile and therefore less likely to erupt and form a blood clot.

Diet 2. Those on Diet 2 saw their homocysteine levels fall 14.6 percent, just slightly better than the Diet 1 results.

Diet 3. Those on the AHA-similar, moderate-fat diet experienced a 9 percent increase in homocysteine levels.

Diet 4. People on the high-protein, high-fat diet saw their homocysteine levels rise 12.4 percent, which was not unexpected.

LIPOPROTEIN (A): THE MOST SENSITIVE MARKER
FOR INFLAMMATION AND LIVER FUNCTION

As discussed in chapter 6, Lp(a) increases the likelihood of blood clots and makes platelets adhere to one another, thus increasingly the likelihood that those clots will increase in size and thus become more dangerous. It is also a major indicator for inflammation and is one of the tests that reveals the health of the liver. Here's how the four diets affected Lp(a) levels.

Diet 1. The people on Diet 1 saw their Lp(a) reduced by 7.4 percent.

Diet 2. Those on Diet 2 saw their Lp(a) levels reduced by 10.8 percent. Finding the reason why Phase 2 had better Lp(a) results will require further study. In any case, any time you get a drop in Lp(a) it means the health of your liver is improving.

Diet 3. Those on the AHA-similar diet saw their Lp(a) levels go up 4.7 percent.

Diet 4. The people who followed the high-protein, high-fat diet experienced a 31 percent increase in Lp(a), which means their risk of blood clots, heart attacks, and strokes went up dramatically.

FIBRINOGEN: HIGH LEVELS MEAN VISCOUS BLOOD, CLOTS, HEART ATTACKS, AND STROKES

Diet 1. Those on Diet 1 experienced an 11 percent reduction in fibrinogen levels.

Diet 2. Those on Diet 2 saw their fibrinogen levels reduced by 6.3 percent.

Diet 3. Those on the AHA-similar moderate-fat diet experienced a 0.6 percent reduction in fibrinogen.

Diet 4. People who followed the high-protein, high-fat diet saw their fibrinogen levels go up 11.9 percent.

What It All Means

One of my motivations for doing the preventive cardiology study was my desire to confirm a whole host of findings that came from an earlier experiment I did in 1999. That study examined the effects of two different diets on people with already existing heart disease (Fleming 2000). My colleagues and I followed 26 people for one year. Both groups received the same medical treatment. Ten of the 26 participants adhered to a high-protein, high-fat diet; 16 followed a high-carbohydrate, low-fat diet. During that year, we monitored the cholesterol, homocysteine, Lp(a), fibrinogen, and C-reactive protein levels of both groups. I also did myocardial perfusion imaging, or nuclear studies, on both groups to measure the amount of blood flowing to their hearts. The results were clear and unequivocal.

After one year on their respective diets, the people on the high-protein diet showed an increase in all the cardiovascular risk factors and a definite progression of their coronary heart disease. Blood tests showed an elevation in cholesterol levels, homocysteine (up 3 percent), lipoprotein (a) (up 106 percent), fibrinogen (up 14 percent), and C-reactive protein (up 61 percent). Myocardial profusion imaging studies revealed a significant decrease in blood flow to the heart for those on the high-protein diet. These people were closer to having a heart attack or stroke than they were before they adopted the high-protein diet.

The group on the high-carb, low-fat diet showed improvement in cardiovascular risk factors and an increase in blood flow to the heart, associated with regression of the atherosclerosis within the coronary arteries. Remarkably, people on the low-fat diet also experienced recovery of heart muscle function that had previously been lost as a result of their advanced heart disease. My research had clearly demonstrated that high-protein diets promote heart disease. On the other hand, a low-fat, high-carbohydrate diet can restore heart function and reverse the underlying illness.

Though the study was small, it was nonetheless a revelation. No one had done such a study on people who ate a high-protein diet, and it contradicted many of the claims made by proponents of such regimens.

High Protein, High Fat Means High Risk

When you increase the risk factors for heart disease, you also raise your chances of contracting other inflammatory illness, such as diabetes, cancer, rheumatoid arthritis, and heart disease. In fact, many studies show that, when people with rheumatoid arthritis adopt vegetarian diets, their arthritis symptoms are eliminated within one year. Plant-based diets that are high in complex carbohydrates, low in animal foods, and low in fat reduce inflammation considerably. This is why they are the best form of medicine for reversing cardiovascular disease and for treating other forms of degenerative illness, including diabetes. A low-fat, plant-based diet is also a powerful form of preventive medicine against the most common cancers.

Don't Let the Weight Loss Fool You

The desperation of people to lose weight has prevented them from seeing what a high price they pay for adopting a high-protein, high-fat diet. These diets do bring about weight loss, by using three weight-loss tools.

First, they are lower in calories than the standard American diet, which by itself will cause weight loss. Second, they restrict carbohydrates so much that your body is thrown into a condition associated with starvation that's known as ketosis, marked by high levels of ketones in the tissues and body fluids. When your body is in ketosis it essentially convinces your brain that there's a famine occurring. Your brain prefers carbohydrates as its primary source of fuel. When you restrict carbohydrates, you prevent the brain from getting the fuel it needs to function. In order to survive, the brain tells the body to turn protein into sugar, a process known as gluconeogenesis. Essentially, that means that you are using protein as your fuel supply. Most of the protein in your body is stored in your muscles, which means you are using muscle mass as your fuel source. That's not a long-term solution, since using your muscles for fuel pretty much ruins any chance you have of gathering food and surviving. Your brain knows this and realizes that it must change its fuel source if you are to survive. So the brain performs another act of magic by ordering the liver to turn stored body fat into ketones, a substance the brain can burn. Now you're burning your own fat, which means you're losing weight.

Once you're in ketosis, your appetite is suppressed—another bit of wisdom from the body that believes it's starving. No point in thinking about food if there is no food. This diminished appetite is the third way these diets can cause weight reduction. All three of these tools also cause significant water loss, which causes even more weight reduction.

None of this is good for your body. It also triggers tremendous cravings for carbohydrates from grains, grain products, and vegetables. You may be losing weight, but your health is declining, and you're experiencing cravings that will only get worse. Eventually you're going to crack and eat a carbohydrate-rich food—most likely a calorically-dense processed food that will take you out of ketosis and start the weight-gaining cycle all over again.

Bone Health

There are other ramifications of high-protein diets, however. Among the most dangerous is the loss of bone mass and the increase in your chances of contracting osteoporosis.

Osteoporosis (literally, "porous bones") affects 10 million Americans, most of them women. As the bones weaken, they become more vulnerable to fracture. About one third of American women will suffer a hip fracture, and approximately 20 percent of those breaks will lead to fatal complications. In all, each year about 1.5 million women suffer a bone break as a result of osteoporosis. At no other time in history has osteoporosis affected more people than it does today.

The reason more women than men get osteoporosis is because women experience a diminution in estrogen production after menopause. The sex hormones—estrogen in women and testosterone in men—are essential for healthy bones.

Bone loss is a natural process. After the age of 35 or so, everyone starts to lose bone mass at a rate of about 1 percent per year. After menopause, women can lose 3 to 5 percent of their bone mass per year. About five years after menopause, that dramatic loss slows to about 1 percent per year. Unfortunately, a woman could have lost a significant amount of bone by that time.

During the past 25 years, we have had the message drummed into our heads that osteoporosis is a disease that results from inadequate calcium intake. We are routinely urged to eat foods that contain calcium, including milk products (those white-mustache ads are as misleading as they are charming), calcium-foritified orange juice, and even antacids that contain calcium, such as Tums. If we judge this educational campaign by our calcium intake, the ads are succeeding admirably. The United States and the Scandinavian countries are among the top calcium consumers in the world. Unfortunately, two other facts about the United States and Sweden are a bit unsettling: we are also among the leaders in bone fractures, especially broken hips. In fact, the United States has the worst hip-fracture rate in the world.

How is it possible, you might ask, that we are eating all this calcium and still suffering from an epidemic of osteoporosis? Well, all those white mustaches aside, calcium, and specifically milk, is not the answer to our osteoporosis epidemic.

"There's no solid evidence that merely increasing the amount of milk in your diet will protect you from breaking a hip or wrist or crushing a backbone in later years," writes Dr. Walter Willett, the head of the Department of Nutrition at Harvard Medical School and author of *Eat, Drink, and Be Healthy: The Harvard Medical School Guide to Healthy Eating.*

How did we come to believe such a thing was possible? A lot of credit for that false belief goes to the National Dairy Council, which, according to the chairperson of the Department of Food Studies at New York University, Marion Nestle, Ph.D., has been the leading source of nutrition information in America.

In her book, *Food Politics: How the Food Industry Influences Nutrition and Health,* Dr. Nestle reveals that the National Dairy Council has been the primary source of nutrition information in the United States. The irony, Dr. Nestle says, is that the dairy industry has succeeded wildly, despite significant scientific evidence supporting concerns about dairy foods.

"As it turns out," Dr. Nestle writes, "nutritionists have collaborated with dairy lobbies to promote the nutritional value of dairy products since the early years of the twentieth century. Recently, however, some scientists have raised doubts about whether dairy foods confer special health benefits. In addition to concerns about lactose intolerance, some question the conventional wisdom that dairy foods protect against osteoporosis or, for that matter, accomplish any public health goals. Others suggest that the hormones, growth factors, and allergenic proteins in dairy foods end up doing more harm than good."

If we clear away the fog that's been created by political and economic interests, we can see very clearly that many lifestyle factors, especially diet and exercise, greatly affect calcium balance and bone strength.

Calcium balance is determined to a great extent by two factors: your calcium intake and the amount of protein you consume. Your body is designed to maintain a balanced pH. This is essential for the health of your blood, organs, and immune system. Animal proteins, which contain an abundance of sulfa-amino acids, are converted in the body to acid. As you eat more animal protein, your acid load increases. Whenever the acid-alkaline balance is thrown off by increased acid levels, the brain signals the bones to release phosphorus and calcium into the bloodstream in order to buffer, or alkalize, the excess acid. This means that the more protein you eat, the higher the acid levels in your blood, and the more phosphorus and calcium your bones will lose.

I like the analogy created by John McDougall, M.D., author of *The Mc-Dougall Program for Women*. He says that eating excess animal protein is the human body's "equivalent of acid rain."

Harvard University's Mark Hegsted, Ph.D., found that when a person's protein intake is doubled, his or her calcium loss also increases by about 50 percent (Hegsted 2001). Very few women can lose that much calcium and still maintain healthy bones.

The ongoing Harvard Nurses Study, in which researchers have been following just over 80,000 women since 1976, has found that women who eat the most protein each day have much higher rates of wrist fractures than women who eat the least protein.

Health authorities, such as the National Academy of Sciences, recommend that Americans eat at least 1,000 mg of calcium per day. Women who are at risk of suffering osteoporosis should consume 1,200 to 1,500 mg of calcium per day, they say. Only in the United States and certain European nations do people consume that much calcium. Ironically, these are also the countries that have the highest rates of osteoporosis.

All that excess milk and calcium may be doing even more harm. The long-term Health Professionals Follow-up Study, which has been following over 50,000 male health professionals since 1986, has found that men who drank two glasses of milk or more per day were nearly two times as likely to develop metastatic prostate cancer than those who drank no milk at all. When the data from this study and others were examined more closely, the researchers found that men who consumed 2,000 mg of calcium a day from food and supplements were three times as likely to develop prostate cancer as those who consumed low amounts of calcium. A study by two Japanese researchers, H. Araki and H. Watanabe, showed that regular milk consumption doubles the risk of prostate enlargement. Daily meat consumption tripled the risk, the researchers found.

Similar patterns have been found in women. Harvard University's Dr. Daniel Cramer and his colleagues found that the sugar in milk, lactose, is broken down into another sugar, called galactose. The body produces enzymes to break down galactose even further. However, as milk consumption increases, the body cannot produce sufficient enzymes to break down and eliminate all the galactose being ingested. This simple sugar injures women's ovaries, research is now suggesting. Some women, who drink greater amounts of milk and appear to be particularly sensitive to the galactose, have three times the rates of ovarian cancer as the national average (Cramer 1989).

Epidemiologists point out that the countries that consume lower amounts of calcium also have the lowest rates of osteoporosis. Indeed, in places like Japan, India, and Singapore, where osteoporosis levels are exceedingly low, calcium intake averages around 300 mg a day. Consistent with worldwide standards, the World Health Organization recommends that men and women consume 400 to 500 mg of calcium per day in order to maintain health, including bone strength.

Another interesting fact is that osteoporosis tends to be lower in countries that consume low levels of dairy foods, or none at all. Writing in the journal *Science*, Dr. Walter Willett stated: "Adult populations with low fracture rates generally consume few dairy products and have low calcium intakes. Milk and other dairy products may not be directly equivalent to calcium from supplements, as these foods contain a substantial amount of protein, which can enhance renal [kidney] calcium losses." Dr. Willett points out that much more research is needed in this area, but a trend has clearly emerged.

The important thing for you to realize is that, in your body, calcium and protein have a kind of see-saw relationship. As protein levels go up, the calcium content of your bones goes down. As protein levels go down, calcium in your bones goes up.

It's worth noting that excess protein and acid levels can injure kidneys and lead to kidney stones.

All of this reveals yet another reason why high-protein diets should be avoided.

Exercise and Your Bones

There are other important factors that either increase or decrease your bone strength, the most important of which is exercise. Believe it or not, bones are much like muscle: the more you use them, the stronger they become. The opposite is also true: sit around and rest your bones and they get weaker and more prone to fracture. The reason is that weight-bearing exercises, including walking, cause bones to break down and rebuild themselves in stronger, denser form. Walking is obviously a weight-bearing exercise; even in comfortable, padded shoes, it involves some degree of shock to the bones, which increases bone breakdown and rebuilding.

In addition to walking, the best exercises for strengthening your bones are various forms of weight training. This can include wrist weights (five-pound weights used while walking can be enough to exercise the wrists, arms, and shoulders) and ankle weights for the legs and ankles. Various types of weight-training exercise machines found in health clubs, YMCAs, and gyms can also be great for building bone density. Exercise physiologists state that it takes about a year of regular weight-bearing exercise to rebuild bone mass. Of course, during that year, you can see tremendous benefit to your muscles and cardiovascular system.

There are numerous other factors that play a role in whether or not you develop osteoporosis. Here are the most important ones.

VITAMIN D

The body needs vitamin D to absorb calcium and maintain bone mass. Vitamin D is fat-soluble, which means that it is stored in the tissues over long periods of time. You can get all the vitamin D you need from about 20 minutes of daily exposure to sunlight—that is, at least in the spring and summer months. Some research shows that people living in cold weather climates may not be getting adequate vitamin D in the winter months, and that a deficiency of the vitamin may be one of the reasons for an increase in osteoporosis and bone fractures. The best advice is to hedge your bets and include vitamin D as part of the multivitamin supplement I recommended.

HORMONES

The primary reason why osteoporosis affects more women than men is the severe reduction in estrogen after menopause. In fact, men do experience osteoporosis, but the incidence in men usually lags behind that of women by about 10 years. Men don't see a significant decline in testosterone until they reach their late fifties or early sixties. The link between diminished estrogen levels and osteoporosis is one of the reasons why doctors have prescribed hormone replacement therapy (HRT). Doctors hoped that by replacing estrogen, bone density would be protected. Unfortunately, recent research has shown that HRT's ability to protect bones has been overestimated. In addition, hormone replacement therapy increases the risk of heart attacks, as well as breast and uterine cancers.

There are alternative medical treatments that can protect bone without putting you at risk for heart disease and cancer. A class of drugs known as bisphosphonates are designed to inhibit the breakdown of bone, thus reducing bone loss. Generic forms of the bisphosphonates include alendronate (Fosamax is a popular brand form of alendronate) and etidronate (Didronel is a widely prescribed brand). Another group of drugs that protect against bone loss are the selective estrogen receptor modulators (SERMs). A generic form is raloxifene (Evista is a common prescription brand).

Of course, I also encourage women to eat soy foods, which contain lots of isoflavones, the plant estrogens that will enhance bone retention and rebuilding.

Excess consumption of alcohol weakens bones and increases the risk of hip fractures. Female alcoholics have much higher rates of hip breaks than nonalcoholics.

PHARMACEUTICAL DRUGS

Prednisone and other drugs known as corticosteroids—commonly prescribed to treat inflammatory disorders such as arthritis, Crohn's disease, and inflammatory bowel syndrome—increase bone loss. Be sure to talk to your doctor if you're currently taking any of these drugs.

SALT

Sodium increases urination and promotes increased loss of calcium through the kidneys. Use salt only in cooking. Never add it at the table.

Bone-Density Tests

Bone-density tests are noninvasive procedures that can tell you whether or not osteoporosis is affecting any of your bones. If so, you and your doctor can design a medical and exercise program that can help you restore the strength and density of any bones that may be weak.

Sources of Calcium

As we saw in chapter 9, there are lots of good plant-based sources of calcium. During Phase 2, you can include sardines (480 mg of calcium per tin), salmon (290 mg of calcium in a 3-ounce serving), mackerel (300 mg in 3 ounces), and herring (250 mg in 3 ounces). Phase 2 includes nuts and seeds, both of which can be sources of calcium. (A third of a cup of almonds contain 130 mg of calcium.) Tofu is a great source, as are the green and leafy vegetables, such as broccoli, kale, collard greens, and mustard greens. Beans provide about 100 mg of calcium per cup. Finally, you can include calcium (250 to 500 mg) as part of your supplement.

* * *

High-protein diets are not an answer, either for your weight or your health. Don't start a program that will increase your risk of heart disease, cancer, and osteoporosis, just because you believe it will cause you to lose weight. Start the Phase 1 program and watch your weight—and all your risk factors for disease—go down fast.

Cancer Is Also an Inflammatory Disease

THE MOST IMPORTANT LESSON YOU should take with you from reading this book is that the damage caused by inflammation is so widespread that it becomes the basis for a whole host of serious illnesses—not just heart disease but also diabetes, high blood pressure, arthritis, brain disorders such as Parkinson's disease and Alzheimer's disease, and even the common cancers. But just as we know that inflammation is the cause of many diseases, we also know how to reduce inflammation and affect the outcome of the illness. That's the second lesson you should take from this book: you can do a great deal to control inflammation and reduce your risk of disease. The third lesson is that you can use the Fleming Program, along with your doctor's advice, to treat any inflammatory illness, including the most dreaded disease of all, cancer.

I have had a long-standing interest in cancer. It is my strong belief that if we reduced inflammation, especially in people with breast and prostate cancers, cancer would be easier to bring under control, if not to defeat entirely.

There are many gentle, natural ways to control inflammation, as I have shown. In fact, given how extremely intractable cancer is to treatment, it seems appropriate that we should use every means possible to defeat this illness.

In the mid-1990s I began to use the Phase 1 and Phase 1a diets, along with soy foods and a soy supplement known as Revival Soy, as an adjunct treatment for breast cancer. This program has yielded many positive results. The diet and soy combination has significantly reduced inflammation of breast tissue in women with breast cancer, and has kept cancers in remission. This includes women who had the breast-cancer gene, known as BrCA1, which dramatically increases a woman's chances of developing breast cancer. Many women who adopted this program had already had numerous recurrences of breast cancer after initial diagnosis. Once on the program, those recurrences stopped and their cancers remained in remission.

The apparent success of a simple, plant-based diet and the addition of soy foods led me to conduct a study of this program with 50 women with breast cancer and inflammation of the breast.

Before these women adopted the program, I performed a kind of SPECT imaging called breast enhanced scintigraphy testing (known as BEST imaging) of each woman's breast tissue. BEST imaging uses nuclear imaging technology to provide extremely precise information on inflammation and cellular changes within the breast. After these scans were performed, I placed the women on the Phase 1 diet and the Revival Soy product and then followed them for six months. At the conclusion of the six-month period, I conducted another round of BEST imaging scans.

The results of the study, which are now undergoing peer review prior to publication, show that all 50 women experienced significant reduction in breast tissue inflammation and decreased cancer activity in the breast. Many of these women also show reduced fibrocystic disease of the breast tissue; at the time of this writing, all remain in remission.

Why the STOP INFLAMMATION NOW! Program Works

There are several scientifically based reasons why this diet and soy combination may have a very powerful effect on cancer. The primary reasons why this program may affect the course of cancer are as follows:

1. The diet is extremely low in fat, especially saturated fat. High-fat diets are associated not only with the onset of cancer but also with the promotion of the disease once it manifests. On the other hand, low-fat diets are associated with prevention of cancer and greater longevity in people with already existing cancers. One of the important benefits of a low-fat diet in the treatment of cancer is that it significantly reduces estrogen levels in women and dihydrotestosterone in men. Both of these sex hormones can serve as promoters of cancer.

2. The diet is low in calories, so it also promotes weight loss. The calorie content of one's diet and weight loss are extremely sensitive and controversial issues for people with cancer, because weight loss is automatically associated with advancing malignancy and wasting. However, research is now showing that women with breast cancer who consume excess calories and are overweight are far more likely to experience recurrence of their disease than those whose diets are low in calories. Once cancer goes into remission and then recurs, it is far more difficult to treat and send back into remission again. There is no doubt, however, that excess calories, overweight, and obesity all reduce a woman's chances of survival. This is especially true in light of the fact that excess calories elevate insulin and create insulin resistance, conditions that support the growth of cancer.

   I believe that weight loss, when it occurs on a nutrient-rich diet, may be a survival strategy by the body. By eliminating excess fat, the body reduces a major source of oxidation and cancer-promoting hormones. It also lowers insulin levels. These physical changes would actually strengthen the body's ability to fight the disease and increase its chances of survival.

3. The diet is composed entirely of plant foods, which means it has an abundance of vitamins, minerals, antioxidants, and phytochemicals. Antioxidants and phytochemicals are associated with strong immune and cancer-fighting systems. Certain phytochemicals appear to fight cancer in several different ways.

4. The diet is rich in fiber. Fiber binds with estrogens and blood cholesterol, and promotes healthy bowel function—all extremely beneficial to people with cancer.

5. The diet includes both soy foods and soy protein, both of which contain isoflavones and other cancer-fighting compounds. Studies consistently

show that the use of soy foods and a whole soy protein inhibit cancer in several ways.

6. The program includes gentle exercise, which is anti-inflammatory, and supplements of folic acid, vitamin B_6, and vitamin B_{12}. One of the most interesting features of some cancers is an elevation in homocysteine levels. A major cause of elevated homocysteine levels is too little folic acid in the diet, which can be seen in anemia (not enough red blood cells), leukemia (wrong types of white blood cells), and cancer. I believe that cancer is a failure of the immunologic system, in part due to deficiencies in folic acid levels, which is revealed by the increase in homocysteine levels. This increase in homocysteine may also be the result of increased dietary intake of methionine (an amino acid found in meat, fish, dairy products, and whole grains), and studies have shown that reducing the amount of methionine available to a cancer (e.g., metastatic breast) makes it more responsive to treatment. Treatment should therefore include giving the patient folic acid, vitamin B_6, and vitamin B_{12} to improve homocysteine levels.

Let's look at these one at a time.

1. The diet is very low in fat.

Dietary fat plays a central role in the onset of cancer, especially cancers of the breast and prostate. But it may also determine how long a person lives once he or she develops cancer. Dr. James Hebert and his coworkers at the University of Massachusetts Medical School in Worcester, Massachusetts, followed 472 women who recently had been diagnosed with breast cancer. The researchers closely analyzed the women's diets, exercise habits, and alcohol and tobacco use, and then followed them for up to 10 years. Hebert and his colleagues found that premenopausal women who regularly ate red meat, bacon, and liver had twice the rate of recurrence than those who abstained from these foods. Premenopausal women who ate margarine and butter had a 67 percent greater chance of recurrence than those who avoided these fats.

A similar pattern exists for men with cancers of the prostate. Diet appears to play a central role in determining whether or not a prostate cancer becomes malignant. Men who have cancerous cells in their prostate and eat high-fat diets have much higher rates of malignant prostate cancer—meaning cancers that spread to other organs, and therefore become much more lethal. On the other hand, men who have cancerous cells in their prostates and who eat low-fat diets are much more likely to have the illness remain confined to the prostate.

Most of these men die in old age, never realizing that they had any disease in the prostate tissue. Autopsy studies of men who died from causes other than cancer—an automobile accident, for example—have shown that 30 percent of American men between the ages of 30 and 40 have cancer cells in their prostate glands. By the time American men reach the age of 50, that number jumps to 40 percent. Compare that to men living in Asian countries, such as Hong Kong, where only 16 percent of men have cancerous cells in their prostates by the age of 45. The same low rates of cancerous cells in the prostate are the rule in other Asian countries.

As long as those cancer cells remain in the prostate, the disease never becomes life-threatening. The men lead normal lives, usually without ever knowing that they had small nests of cancer in their prostate glands. However, many more Western men, those living in the United States and Europe, see their latent prostate cancers become full-blown metastases than men who live in Asia. Swedish men, who typically eat a diet rich in fat and processed foods, are eight times more likely to see their latent prostate cancers become full-blown metastases.

The Asian diet is essentially a plant-based diet: it's low in animal foods and fat, and rich in vegetables and grains. Contrast that with the standard American diet, which is rich in meat, dairy products, eggs, and poultry.

Why would fat consumption play a role in the onset and promotion of breast and prostate cancers? Because the fat content of these foods dramatically increases sex hormones, which in turn serve as fuels for cancer.

Dietary fat raises hormone levels in both sexes—estrogen in women and dihydrotestosterone, the hormone responsible for sperm maturation, in men. The body's fat cells produce estrogen. The more fat in the diet, the higher a woman's estrogen levels tend to be. The same is true for dihydrotestosterone, which causes swelling of the prostate and is associated with greater risk of prostate cancer in men. High fat consumption is a major reason why both estrogen and testosterone become imbalanced.

In healthy women, estrogen levels rise during ovulation, the period when a woman's body prepares for pregnancy, and fall just before and during menstruation. When estrogen surges, breast and uterine tissues become inflamed and sensitive. High estrogen levels are among the causes of uterine bleeding, premenstrual syndrome (PMS), ovarian and fibroid cysts, early menarche, and late menopause.

When excessively high estrogen levels are maintained over time, the hormone-sensitive tissues become chronically inflamed and painful. Inside the breasts, milk and lymph ducts can become blocked, scarred, and swollen. As these tissues become inflamed, blood and lymph circulation within the breast becomes impaired. This increases oxidation and the accumulation of waste products within the breast tissue. Under these conditions, many cells die, but some mutate and become cancerous.

Once a cancer manifests, these conditions actually promote its growth. Estrogen is a mitogen, meaning it induces mitosis, or cell division, and can therefore fuel the growth of cancer cells. An estrogen- and oxidant-rich environment is the perfect host for cancer. Under these conditions, a few mutated cells can turn into a forest fire, as it were.

A similar process occurs in men. High-fat diets raise dihydrotestosterone levels, which in turn cause prostate tissue to become inflamed and swollen. Circulation of blood, oxygen, and lymph is diminished. Some of the cells in the prostate can become cancerous. This does not necessarily mean trouble, however, unless those cancer cells spread to other parts of the body, or metastasize. Then the illness can be fatal. This is the reason we see greater mortality among women and men on high-fat diets: these diets fuel the cancer and make it much more difficult to treat.

A study done at Harvard University's School of Public Health by Dr. Edward Giovannucci and his coworkers showed that men with advanced prostate cancer had a higher consumption of saturated fat and omega-6 fatty acids than men who did not have prostate cancer. The foods that were strongly associated with advanced prostate cancers were bacon, creamy salad dressing, butter, and red meat (Giovannucci 1993).

Several studies have shown that low-fat and high-fiber diets reduce the levels of dihydrotestosterone and may improve survival rates in men with prostate cancer.

The bottom line: A diet low in fat can serve as both a preventive measure and an important form of treatment for already existing cancer.

2. The diet is low in calories but rich in nutrients.

Researchers have consistently found that overweight is associated with an elevated risk of cancer. Conversely, weight loss has been found to reduce a woman's chances of contracting breast cancer.

A study done by Dr. Regina Ziegler of the National Institutes of Health showed that weight loss, especially in women in their forties and fifties, significantly reduces the risk of breast cancer. Dr. Ziegler and her colleagues followed 1,563 women, 966 of whom had recently been diagnosed with breast cancer and 597 of whom had not developed the disease. The scientists had the women fill out a questionnaire to provide information on how much they weighed at each decade of life and then divided the women up into five groups depending on their weights. The women who weighed the most were twice as likely to develop breast cancer as those in the lowest-weight group. That was not particularly surprising, since it merely confirmed other studies. What was surprising, though, was that the women who had shed excess weight in their forties and fifties had decreased their risk of getting breast cancer by 50 percent (Ziegler 1996). The reason weight loss played such an important role in the reduction of risk was because it lowered estrogen levels, the researchers said.

But there may be more to weight loss than a reduction in estrogen levels. As weight falls, so too do insulin levels. At the same time, cells become more sensitive to insulin, which means the pancreas does not have to produce as much insulin to maintain glucose metabolism. Research has shown that, like estrogen, insulin can act as a mitogen, or fuel, for cancer cells. The higher the insulin levels, the more cancer cells and tumors thrive. Excess calories and weight ensure higher insulin levels. Conversely, weight loss reduces insulin and insulin resistance and thus eliminates one of the more important fuels for malignancy.

ANY MEASURES THAT LOWER RISK MAY ALSO BE EFFECTIVE AS A FORM OF TREATMENT

It's very important to keep in mind that the very factors that cause cancer in the first place also promote its growth once it manifests. Women with high estrogen levels not only have a greater chance of getting cancer but also have a much reduced chance of survival if cancer develops. The drug tamoxifen is used to lower estrogen effect and increase a woman's chances of going into remission. Overweight increases estrogen, which is one reason why it reduces survival.

Dr. Hebert and his team at the University of Massachusetts found that premenopausal women with breast cancer experienced a 45 percent increase in the risk of recurrence for each 1,000 daily calories consumed above their ideal caloric levels.

Excess calorie consumption and overweight combine to form the basis for high insulin and insulin resistance, a condition referred to as syndrome X. Many researchers now believe that syndrome X plays a major role in the onset of breast cancer and can also create the preconditions for prostate cancer.

Recently, UCLA's James Barnard and his colleagues reported that men with prostate cancer who followed a low-fat diet and who exercised regularly experienced a dramatic drop in insulin levels and insulin-like growth factor I, or IGF-I (described in chapter 6), both of which are fuels for cancer. At the same time, these men produced more of a substance that binds with hormone and helps eliminate it from the body. All of these conditions helped improve the chances of survival among these men (Barnard 2002).

Barnard's study suggests that prostate cancer may be the result of insulin-resistance syndrome, or syndrome X.

The researchers found yet another intriguing reaction in the men on the low-fat diet and exercise program. The cancer cells in their bodies started to die, a process known as apoptosis. Apoptosis is a normal, necessary function of cells, and the aberrant inhibition or initiation of apoptosis contributes to many diseases, including cancer.

One of the more remarkable characteristics of cancer cells is that they are virtually immortal. Not only don't they die, but they change so rapidly that they become increasingly resistant to treatment. Researchers have been trying to find ways to trigger apoptosis, or cell suicide, in cancer cells. Cancer-cell death doesn't happen in environments where cancer cells thrive. In fact, just the opposite happens. The cancer cells mutate more rapidly in environments that are rich with oxidants, high glucose, and insulin, all of which support the life of cancer.

Barnard created an environment that was exactly the opposite: one that was low in insulin, low in glucose, low in oxidants, and high in antioxidants.

This environment was antagonistic to cancer cells. Lo and behold, the cancer cells started to die. It may be that without environmental supports, and in the presence of a nutrient-rich, antioxidant-rich blood supply, cancer cells may suddenly start to experience apoptosis.

I believe the successful treatment of cancer requires three conditions: first, eliminate angiogenesis (growth of new blood vessels) *and* their attachment to the cancer cells. Doing one without the other will not work. In other words, cause a "cancer attack" in the same way a heart attack occurs by depriving the cancer cells of the necessary oxygen and nutrients they need to survive. Second, enhance the function of the immune system of the body through diet, Foltx, et cetera, so the body can deal with the problem directly, and, finally, eliminate or remove the offending agents taken into the body that promoted the development of the cancer to begin with.

As we know, health is improved on diets that are nutrient-rich but low in calories. The bottom line is eat a nutrient-rich diet and lower your weight as a means of prevention and treatment of cancer.

3. A plant-based diet is rich in vitamins, minerals, antioxidants, and important phytochemicals that help fight cancer.

Dr. Hebert's study found that postmenopausal women who ate an additional 100 mg of vitamin C per day—the amount found in a cup of broccoli—experienced a 43 percent reduction in the risk of breast-cancer recurrence.

At the Fred Hutchinson Cancer Research Center in Seattle, researchers found that men who ate at least three servings of vegetables per day had half the risk of developing prostate cancer than men who failed to eat those three daily servings. Cruciferous vegetables were found to be the most protective. Cruciferous vegetables include broccoli, cabbage, collard greens, kale, and mustard greens. Included in that family are sauerkraut and cole slaw, both made from cabbage. Watercress, while not a cruciferous vegetable, is also an excellent choice.

"When we compared relative potency, vegetables from the cruciferous family, like broccoli and cabbage, reduced the risk even further," said Dr. Alan Kristal, one of the researchers involved in the Seattle-area study. The scientists rigorously examined the eating habits of 1,230 men between the ages of 40 and 64. Overall vegetable consumption provided strong protection against prostate cancer, but the cruciferous vegetables were the most effective.

"The bottom line is that if you eat a lot of vegetables, you can cut your risk of prostate cancer by about 45 percent," Dr. Kristal said in the Fred Hutchinson Cancer Research Center newsletter (available at the Fred Hutchinson Cancer Research Center.com website). "And if some of those vegetables are from the cruciferous family, like broccoli and cabbage, you may reduce your risk even further."

In chapter 9, I described many of the health-promoting and cancer-fighting substances in vegetables, including sulforanphane, a substance that promotes detoxification of the blood and tissues and helps to fight cancer. Another is the chemical known as phenethyl isothiocyanate (PEITC), which may inhibit the emergence of lung tumors in animals that have been bred to create cancerous tumors. Indoles and bioflavonoids are other substances that are abundant in many vegetables and grains and also help to fight cancer. And then there are the antioxidants, carotenoids, and phytochemicals. Cancer thrives in an oxidant-rich environment. Antioxidants, on the other hand, reduce and sometimes stop oxidation. They also boost immune function, promote the cancer-fighting systems, and protect healthy cells from mutation. Carotenoids and phytochemicals have their own cancer-fighting properties.

Vegetables, grains, and fruits are abundant in cancer-protective and cancer-fighting substances. In fact, the more we discover about the potency of these substances, the greater our responsibility becomes to encourage people with cancer to eat a diet rich in plant foods as part of an effective cancer treatment program.

4. Eating fiber-rich foods balances hormones and promotes healthy elimination.

There are two ways to drop estrogen and dihydrotestosterone levels rapidly and, in the process, affect the course of breast and prostate cancers: dramatically reduce fat and increase fiber.

Fiber binds with hormones and helps eliminate them through the bowel. A study published in the *New England Journal of Medicine* (1982) showed that vegetarian women who eat high-fiber diets eliminate two to three times more estrogen in their feces than nonvegetarians.

Another study, reported in the scientific journal *Oncologist*, showed that a high-fiber, low-fat diet lowered estrogen levels in a group of postmeno-pausal women by 50 percent (McTiernan 2003). Cutting estrogen levels in half can have an astounding impact on health. Researchers have shown that a 17 percent reduction of estrogen can reduce the risk of breast cancer four- to fivefold, according to a report published in the *Journal of the National Cancer Institute* (Toniolo 1995).

A high-fiber diet also changes the intestinal flora, which in turn change hormonal balance. People on meat-centered diets tend to have high levels of bacteria that produce estrogen-like compounds. These bacteria also allow es- trogens to circulate in the body more than once. In health, all estrogen is chemically tagged by the liver and prevented from being reabsorbed by the small intestine, to ensure that old estrogen doesn't keep circulating while new estrogen is being produced. That would surely drive up estrogen to dan- gerously high levels. However, the bacteria in the intestines of people who are on meat- and dairy-based diets remove that protein tag from the estrogen, which means that the estrogen can be reabsorbed and added to the body's overall estrogen load.

Finally, a high-fiber diet promotes healthy bowel elimination, which is the primary way the body rids itself of excess hormones. By binding with hor- mones and promoting bowel elimination, fiber efficiently rids the body of ex- cess hormones that can cause disease.

Anyone concerned about hormone-driven cancers would be well advised to go on a high-fiber diet.

5. Soy foods and soy protein protect against breast and prostate cancers.

It's no overstatement to say that soybeans and soy products have suddenly burst upon the nutrition landscape as potential superfoods. Two forms of re- search have fueled this awareness of the powers of soy. The first are epide- miological studies that showed that people who eat high amounts of soy foods—namely Asians—have surprisingly low rates of cancer, especially can- cers of the breast and prostate. The second is the relatively recent discovery of a whole host of substances in soybeans that have cancer-fighting proper- ties. The most celebrated of these are substances called isoflavones and, specifically, the isoflavones genistein and daidzein. Genistein has the ability to block the formation of blood vessels to tumors. Like all other tissues, cancerous tumors need a blood supply in order to survive. Genistein's ability to block that blood supply, a talent known as anti-angiogenesis, surprised and excited researchers, because it suggested potentially new ways of treating cancer. Since that time, a great deal of research has been done on soy foods, soy proteins, and the isolated soy isoflavones. Much of that research has revealed a whole host of other anticancer properties in soy foods.

In addition to their anti-angiogenetic effects, soy isoflavones act like plant estrogens, and are considerably milder than those produced by the human body. The human body produces three types of estrogen: estradiol, which has been shown to have cancer-promoting characteristics; estrone, which may also promote cancer; and estriol, which is the mildest of the three and, studies show, does not appear to trigger the cancer process. Like human estrogens, plant estrogens bind to the estrogen receptor sites on cells and essentially substitute for the stronger, more disease-promoting hormones produced by the body. In effect, the plant estrogens, also known as phytoestrogens, do the same job as the body's estrogens, but in a milder, gentler way. We now believe that these phytoestrogens take up residence on the cell and protect it from the cancer-promoting effects of estradiol and estrone.

The estrogen-like properties of these isoflavones have also caused them to be seen as a potential substitute for HRT—specifically, as chemicals that may protect women from bone loss after menopause. Some studies suggest that women who eat foods rich in soy isoflavones may have stronger bones than women who do not eat these foods. Other research has shown that women whose diets contain a steady supply of soy foods have milder menopausal symptoms than those who do not eat soybean products. In addition to these protective benefits, soy foods are loaded with antioxidants and other phytochemicals that may have their own independent anticancer properties. The point to keep in mind is that soy foods appear to protect against cancer, and even attack cancer cells and tumors, in a variety of ways.

Still, concerns have been raised that soy foods may promote already existing estrogen-sensitive cancers in some women. Some scientists theorize that the weak estrogenic effects of soy foods could fuel cancers, just as HRT and naturally occurring estrogens do. These scientists argue that postmenopausal women with cancer may be especially vulnerable to plant estrogen. The reason is that women who are past menopause have diminished estrogen levels in their bodies. The introduction of soy foods into their diets might present a new source of estrogens that could act as a fuel for cancers in these women. Scientists argue that this might be especially true for women with cancers that are estrogen receptor–positive—cancers that are stimulated by estrogen.

I am not persuaded by the small number of laboratory studies that appear to support these findings. Here's why.

When all the studies done on soy foods—that is, all the research done on humans, on animals, and in test tubes—are taken into account, over 94 percent of the studies have shown that soy foods inhibit the growth of cancer. In addition, all the human research has shown that soy foods protect people from cancers, even people whose cancers are estrogen receptor–positive.

The only studies that contradict this conclusion are those that have been done in vitro, meaning in a test tube or dish. These studies haven not been done with whole soy foods, but with isolated isoflavones. Researchers have extracted purified genistein from soybeans and then artificially introduced it to a line of cancer cells in a test tube and watched what the genistein would do to the cancer. In some cases, these cancers have grown.

There are numerous problems with this kind of research. First, it does not reflect what happens in nature, meaning what takes place when a human being eats a soy food or a whole-soy product. When people eat a soy product, they consume a whole food that includes a range of anticancer compounds. We do not know how these compounds interact with each other, or which ones are the most powerful. Genistein is an important substance, but it may be powerless, or even toxic, without other chemicals found in soybeans. By taking genistein out of the soybean, we may have altered it irrevocably, and then introduced this artificial chemical into a line of cancer cells. That chemical bears no resemblance to food found in nature.

However, no study—not even those done in test tubes—has shown that isolated isoflavones change normal cells into cancerous ones.

Scientists are well aware that isolated chemicals taken from plants do not behave in a test tube in the same way that they act in the human body when they are consumed as food. The anticancer chemicals in, say, broccoli or other cruciferous vegetables, do not have nearly the same effect when they are extracted from the broccoli as they do when a person eats the whole broccoli spear. In fact, many of these anticancer compounds found in food actually promote cancer when they are extracted from the food and applied to a line of cancer cells in a test tube. Scientists routinely dismiss these studies, because they know that plant chemicals behave differently when they are removed from the whole plant—just as genistein behaves differently when it is extracted from the soybeans and added to cancer cells.

Revival Soy is ground-up soybeans that have been dried and made into a powder that can be combined with water or fruit juice. It contains 180 mg of isoflavones, including genistein, daidzein, and glycitein; 100 mg of saponins, a phytochemical that has anticancerous properties; and L-arginine, a powerful antioxidant that also has been shown to fight cancer.

In addition to my own study on Revival Soy mentioned earlier, other research has found that the Revival Soy product triggered apoptosis, or programmed cell death, in breast-cancer patients.

In 1999 the FDA reviewed all the data related to soy foods and cancer, including in vitro studies using isolated isoflavones, and determined that there is no basis to support the claim that soy foods promote cancer, even in women with estrogen-sensitive cancers.

The question naturally arises: Why would anyone interested in researching soy foods isolate a single chemical in a food that contains a multiplicity of substances, many of which have already been shown to have anticancerous properties? The answer is simple: economic gain. Pharmaceutical companies are eager to isolate a single active ingredient so that they can patent and market a controllable product. Unfortunately, when economic incentives drive scientific inquiry, you can easily get a distorted picture of the truth.

6. Exercise has been shown to protect both men and women from cancer.

Exercise reduces weight, lowers estrogen levels, lowers insulin, increases insulin sensitivity, boosts immune function, strengthens the cancer-fighting systems, and reduces inflammation. No medication can do all of that for you.

In study after study, exercise has been shown to protect against all the common cancers, heart disease, diabetes, high blood pressure, and digestive disorders. Exercise is especially powerful when it comes to protecting women from breast cancer.

A study done by Italian researchers, the results of which were published in the *Journal of the National Cancer Institute* in 1998, found that about one third of breast cancers can be avoided by drinking only small amounts of alcohol, eating foods rich in vitamin E and beta-carotene, namely plant foods, and exercising regularly.

Dr. Maura Mezzetti of the European Institute of Oncology in Milan and her coworkers studied 2,569 women with breast cancer and compared them to 2,588 matched controls, or women without cancer. Both groups provided extensive information on their health habits, diets, and exercise patterns for the previous two years before diagnosis.

The researchers found that, in premenopausal women, 43 percent of breast-cancer cases were associated with high alcohol consumption and low physical activity. In postmenopausal women, 41 percent of cases were associated with excess body weight and low physical activity.

Regular exercise reduces or eliminates the underlying conditions that combine to form syndrome X. Since syndrome X can lead to both breast and prostate cancer, the reduction or elimination of these symptoms can be a formula for prevention of both diseases. It can even help you if you are currently battling either breast or prostate cancer.

Some studies show that an hour of vigorous exercise may increase your lifespan by two years. Take a 20- to 30-minute walk four to six times a week. Engage in some form of aerobic activity that you enjoy and find emotionally rewarding—a game, dancing, or a martial art, for example. Exercise is good for body, mind, and soul. Coupled with the Fleming STOP INFLAMMATION NOW! diet, it can change your life for the better, no matter what your current state of health may be.

If you decide to follow the Fleming Program, I strongly urge you to continue to be treated by your medical doctor. This program is not meant to be a substitute for medical treatment. Medical treatment remains the primary source of health care for serious illness, especially cancer. Tell your doctor that you are using this program so that he or she can follow more closely the effects of the STOP INFLAMMATION NOW! Program on your disease.

Inflammation Is the Problem
Diet and Exercise Are the Solution

The typical Western diet and lifestyle that currently shape our lives have turned our immune defenses against us. The very system that has sustained human existence for nearly 2 million years is now the basis for our destruction. In the past 50 years, we have turned nature on its head. Why? Because we insist on eating foods that nature never intended us to eat. The poisons in those processed foods have transformed our bodies into breeding grounds for disease. The immune system was designed to defeat both the conditions that support disease as well as the illnesses themselves. Unfortunately, most of us today feed those disease-causing conditions every day of our lives. The consequence is that our immune systems must overwork, and, in their extreme efforts to keep us alive, they release inflammatory reactions that contribute to premature illness and death.

The miracle of the human body is that many, if not all, of these conditions can be turned around. Health can be restored. We can cool the fires of inflammation simply by eliminating its causes and adding food substances that help the immune system do its job. In this book, I have tried to provide a clear formula for the significant reduction of inflammation and the recovery of health. Adopt the Fleming Program and watch your life change.

If you follow this plan, you will find yourself losing weight. Your cholesterol, triglyceride, homocysteine, Lp(a), fibrinogen, growth factors, and leukotrienes can all fall into the normal ranges. Allow your doctor to follow your progress as you reduce all the risk factors that form the basis for heart disease, diabetes, and cancer. As your health improves, your physician may want to alter any medication you are currently taking.

As your numbers change, your daily experience of life will very likely be radically transformed as well. As you feel stronger, more vital and alive, you will start to see changes in what you think is possible to achieve in your life. And all of this flows from these simple foods—vegetables, fruits, and whole grains, the foods we were designed to eat.

13

Menus

*

IN THIS CHAPTER I PROVIDE THREE
weeks of menus each for the Phase 1 and Phase 2 diets. Both diets present a
wide variety of foods. Every entrée listed has a corresponding recipe in the
next chapter. The only exceptions are the self-explanatory meals, such as
fresh fruit or some cooked-fruit combinations. I also provide recipes for all
the dressings and sauces recommended for your Phase 1 vegetables and
beans, and your Phase 2 whole grains, vegetables, beans, and pasta dishes.
The recipe chapter also provides numerous suggestions for ways to prepare
meals and sauces quickly.

There are several types of drinks to choose from with each meal. These
include clean, pure water (choose spring water whenever possible); various
kinds of herbal teas, such as chamomile; black and green tea; and coffee substitutes, such as Pero and others made from chicory and barley.

I recommend that you eat fresh fruit and vegetable salads throughout
the Phase 1 program. Fruit salad may contain apples, bananas, berries, canta-

loupe, cherries, green and red grapes, honeydew melon, oranges, pears, peaches, and tangerines. Whenever you make vegetable salads, include dark-green lettuce and lots of different vegetables, including broccoli, cauliflower, red and green peppers, Brussels sprouts, and tomatoes. Salads are especially delicious and satisfying when you include beans, such as chickpeas or pinto beans.

Here are menu ideas for the Phase 1 and Phase 2 diets. (Recipes for the dishes shown in capital letters are given in chapter 14. To help you quickly locate these recipes, see the "Index of Recipes" at the end of this section that lists in alphabetical order all recipes included in both the Phase 1 and Phase 2 diets.) Enjoy!

The Phase 1 Diet

WEEK ONE

* Sunday *

BREAKFAST	LUNCH	DINNER
Stewed prunes, figs, and raisins, garnished with ground and roasted flaxseeds	CHINESE-STYLE VEGETABLES, garnished with flaxseeds Salad with chickpeas, tomato, and Bermuda onion, and ORANGE DRESSING	BAKED SWEET POTATO ROOT STEW STEAMED GREENS (watercress and broccoli) Unsweetened applesauce

* Monday *

BREAKFAST	LUNCH	DINNER
MISO SOUP Stewed apples and pears, topped with roasted and ground-up flaxseeds	STEAMED GREENS (asparagus), garnished with grated garlic and lemon Salad with carrots, cucumber, and chickpeas, and ORANGE DRESSING	RED LENTIL SOUP STEAMED GREENS (collards) CHINESE-STYLE VEGETABLES SCRAMBLED TOFU STEWED PEACHES

* Tuesday *

BREAKFAST	LUNCH	DINNER
Large fresh fruit salad of cantaloupe, blueberries, apples, bananas, and oranges	Vegetable soup ROOT STEW Salad with tofu, Bermuda onion, and raw broccoli, and LEMON DRESSING Fruit dessert	GREEN LENTIL SOUP WITH POTATO RATATOUILLE STEAMED GREENS (asparagus) RUTABAGA PICKLES

* Wednesday *

BREAKFAST	LUNCH	DINNER
SQUASH SOUP Fresh fruit salad	ADUKI BEANS Steamed kale, broccoli, and onions RUTABAGA PICKLES Fresh fruit	Salad with broccoli and cauliflower, and TOFU DRESSING CHINESE-STYLE VEGETABLES BOILED CARROTS AND PARSNIPS APPLES WITH APRICOT SAUCE

* Thursday *

BREAKFAST	LUNCH	DINNER
Fresh fruit salad	RED LENTIL SOUP Salad with broccoli, cauliflower, and chopped and steamed tofu, and LEMON DRESSING	BAKED SWEET POTATO OR YAM WATER-SAUTÉED CARROTS, ONIONS, AND SUMMER SQUASH STEAMED GREENS (mustard)

* Friday *

BREAKFAST	LUNCH	DINNER
Fresh fruit salad, garnished with flaxseeds	Salad with chickpeas, carrots, and cauliflower STEAMED GREENS (broccoli) RUTABAGA PICKLES Sliced kiwi fruit and bananas	PINTO BEANS SQUASH SOUP CHINESE-STYLE VEGETABLES DAIKON RADISH WITH SHOYU STEWED PEACHES

* Saturday *

BREAKFAST	LUNCH	DINNER
Vegetable soup Stewed prunes, figs, and raisins, with flaxseeds	BAKED SWEET POTATO OR YAM Salad with broccoli, black beans, and carrots, and ORANGE DRESSING RATATOUILLE Apple	RED LENTIL SOUP STEAMED GREENS (Brussels sprouts and kale) DAIKON RADISH SALAD SCRAMBLED TOFU APPLE-LEMON KANTEN

WEEK TWO

* Sunday *

BREAKFAST	LUNCH	DINNER
Fresh fruit salad, garnished with flaxseeds	Boiled squash, parsnips, and carrots Steamed watercress, carrots, and tofu medley, with ORANGE DRESSING	GREEN LENTIL SOUP WITH POTATO CHINESE-STYLE VEGETABLES STEAMED GREENS APPLES WITH APRICOT SAUCE

* Monday *

BREAKFAST	LUNCH	DINNER
MISO SOUP Steamed collard greens and carrots Fresh fruit salad	RATATOUILLE SCRAMBLED TOFU Salad with broccoli, red onions, and carrots, and TOFU DRESSING Fresh fruit	RED LENTIL SOUP PLAIN BAKED POTATO Steamed collards, carrots, and parsnips Fresh fruit dessert

* Tuesday *

BREAKFAST	LUNCH	DINNER
Fresh fruit salad with flaxseeds	Vegetable soup Salad with three vegetables of your choice, and ORANGE DRESSING CHINESE-STYLE VEGETABLES	GREEN LENTIL SOUP WITH POTATO STEAMED GREENS (asparagus) RUTABAGA PICKLES BOILED CARROTS AND PARSNIPS

* Wednesday *

BREAKFAST	LUNCH	DINNER
Cooked fruit combo, garnished with flaxseeds	ROOT STEW STEAMED GREENS (kale) ADUKI BEANS Fresh fruit	Salad with chickpeas, onions, and carrots, and TOFU DRESSING STEAMED GREENS (Brussels sprouts) RUTABAGA PICKLES BAKED SQUASH APPLE-LEMON KANTEN

* Thursday *

BREAKFAST	LUNCH	DINNER
SCRAMBLED TOFU	RED LENTIL SOUP Salad with broccoli, cauliflower, and scallions, and LEMON DRESSING Fresh fruit	PLAIN BAKED POTATO STEAMED GREENS (mustard) CHINESE-STYLE VEGETABLES APPLES WITH APRICOT SAUCE

* Friday *

BREAKFAST	LUNCH	DINNER
Fresh fruit salad, garnished with flaxseeds	BAKED SWEET POTATO OR YAM STEAMED GREENS (kale) RUTABAGA PICKLES Fresh fruit	Baked tofu with ORANGE DRESSING BAKED SWEET POTATO OR YAM BOILED CARROTS AND PARSNIPS Salad with chickpeas, cauliflower, and broccoli, and dressing of your choice Fresh fruit salad

* Saturday *

BREAKFAST	LUNCH	DINNER
SCRAMBLED TOFU Fresh fruit	BAKED SWEET POTATO OR YAM RATATOUILLE STEAMED GREENS (Brussels sprouts) Fresh fruit	PINTO BEANS SQUASH SOUP Steamed cauliflower and broccoli APPLES WITH APRICOT SAUCE

WEEK THREE

* Sunday *

BREAKFAST	LUNCH	DINNER
Stewed apples, pears, and berries, garnished with flaxseeds	BAKED SWEET POTATO OR YAM Salad with broccoli, cauliflower, and tofu, and LEMON DRESSING Fresh fruit	MISO SOUP BOILED BEANS (black), cooked with onions, carrots, and tomatoes Steamed kale, collard greens, and onions

* Monday *

BREAKFAST	LUNCH	DINNER
Stewed prunes, figs, and raisins, garnished with flaxseeds Tea or grain coffee	ADUKI BEANS Salad with cucumbers, Bermuda onions, and tomatoes, and ORANGE DRESSING PLAIN BAKED POTATO Fresh fruit Spring water, tea, or grain coffee	ROOT STEW RATATOUILLE STEAMED GREENS (broccoli) SCRAMBLED TOFU Fresh fruit salad Spring water, tea, or grain coffee

* Tuesday *

BREAKFAST	LUNCH	DINNER
Cooked-fruit combo Tea or grain coffee	BAKED SWEET POTATO OR YAM Salad with chickpeas, broccoli, and Bermuda onions, and TOFU DRESSING Fresh fruit Tea, grain coffee, or spring water	GREEN LENTIL SOUP WITH POTATO STEAMED GREENS (Brussels sprouts) Salad with tomato, onions, peppers, and carrots Tea, grain coffee, or spring water

* Wednesday *

BREAKFAST	LUNCH	DINNER
SQUASH SOUP Fresh fruit Tea or grain coffee substitute	Vegetable soup PLAIN BAKED POTATO with salsa Salad with carrots and cauliflower, and LEMON DRESSING Fresh fruit	RED LENTIL SOUP DAIKON RADISH WITH SHOYU Steamed kale and carrots RATATOUILLE Fresh fruit

* Thursday *

BREAKFAST	LUNCH	DINNER
SCRAMBLED TOFU	Vegetable soup BAKED SWEET POTATO OR YAM STEAMED GREENS (kale) Salad with raw broccoli and chickpeas, and ORANGE DRESSING Fresh fruit Tea, grain coffee, or spring water	BOILED BEANS (black) cooked with red peppers, onions, and garlic BOILED CARROTS AND PARSNIPS CHINESE-STYLE VEGETABLES STEAMED GREENS (watercress) APPLES WITH APRICOT SAUCE Spring water, tea, or grain coffee

* Friday *

BREAKFAST	LUNCH	DINNER
STEWED PEACHES Tea or grain coffee	SQUASH SOUP Salad with grated turnips, scallions, and mushrooms, and TOFU DRESSING Fresh fruit Tea, grain coffee, or spring water	RED LENTIL SOUP PLAIN BAKED POTATO with salsa RATATOUILLE STEAMED GREENS (broccoli) APPLE-LEMON KANTEN

* Saturday *

BREAKFAST	LUNCH	DINNER
Stewed prunes, figs, and raisins, garnished with flaxseeds Tea or grain coffee	Vegetable soup ADUKI BEANS CHINESE-STYLE VEGETABLES Fresh fruit Spring water, grain coffee, or tea	GREEN LENTIL SOUP WITH POTATO ROOT STEW STEAMED GREENS (kale) RUTABAGA PICKLES SCRAMBLED TOFU Fresh fruit Beverage

The Phase 2 Diet

WEEK ONE

* Sunday *

BREAKFAST	LUNCH	DINNER
QUINOA PORRIDGE	BUCKWHEAT AND BOWS	MISO SOUP
STEWED PEACHES	Salad with tomatoes, broccoli, and onions, and SESAME-LEMON DRESSING	FRIED RICE WITH SHRIMP AND VEGETABLES
	Fresh fruit	CHINESE-STYLE VEGETABLES
		STEAMED GREENS (Brussels sprouts)
		ROOT STEW
		Fresh fruit

* Monday *

BREAKFAST	LUNCH	DINNER
OATMEAL	SQUASH SOUP	Vegetable soup
Fresh fruit	MARINATED CHICKPEA SALAD	Linguini with green vegetables and tomato sauce
	CABBAGE WITH CUMIN	Salad with three vegetables, and VINAIGRETTE DRESSING
		BLUEBERRY CRISP

* Tuesday *

BREAKFAST	LUNCH	DINNER
QUINOA PORRIDGE	BROILED WHITE FISH	SHIITAKE AND BARLEY SOUP
Fresh fruit	RUTABAGA PICKLES	BOILED BROWN RICE
	STEAMED GREENS (kale)	LUSCIOUS LEEKS
		MARINATED VEGETABLES
		Sautéed broccoli and cauliflower
		BLUEBERRY CRISP

* Wednesday *

BREAKFAST	LUNCH	DINNER
OATMEAL	UDON NOODLES IN BROTH	Broiled skinless chicken
Fresh fruit	SAUTÉED GREENS	ROOT STEW
Tea or grain coffee	MARINATED CHICKPEA SALAD	PRESSED CUCUMBER SALAD
	Fresh fruit	STEAMED GREENS (broccoli)
	Tea, grain coffee, or spring water	Tea, grain coffee, or spring water

* Thursday *

BREAKFAST	LUNCH	DINNER
Two-egg-white omelette with onions, mushrooms, tomatoes, and broccoli Tea or grain coffee	COLD SOBA NOODLES WITH GINGER-SESAME SAUCE STEAMED GREENS (watercress) Beverage	RED LENTIL SOUP PRESSURE-COOKED BROWN RICE, served with SCALLION, RED PEPPER, AND SESAME-SEED CONDIMENT SAUTÉED GREENS (mustard) BAKED SQUASH STEWED PEACHES Beverage

* Friday *

BREAKFAST	LUNCH	DINNER
MILLET WITH VEGETABLES Fresh fruit Tea or grain coffee	Vegetable soup ROASTED POTATOES Dark green salad with carrots, chickpeas, and tofu, and MISO DRESSING Fresh fruit Beverage	BAKED SALMON DAIKON RADISH SALAD SAUTÉED GREENS (asparagus) RATATOUILLE Toasted sunflower seeds with raisins Fresh fruit

* Saturday *

BREAKFAST	LUNCH	DINNER
Fresh fruit salad Tea or grain coffee	Vegetable soup MACARONI AND BEAN SALAD STEAMED GREENS (watercress) Fresh fruit	BROILED WHITEFISH SAUTÉED GREENS (collards) BAKED SWEET POTATO OR YAM WILD RICE PILAF APPLE-LEMON KANTEN

WEEK TWO

* Sunday *

BREAKFAST	LUNCH	DINNER
SCRAMBLED TOFU Fresh fruit	WILD RICE PILAF STEAMED GREENS (kale and collards) BAKED SWEET POTATO OR YAM Fresh fruit salad	COLD SOBA NOODLES WITH GINGER-SESAME SAUCE SAUTÉED CARROTS, ONIONS, AND SUMMER SQUASH ROASTED POTATOES STEAMED GREENS (broccoli)

* Monday *

BREAKFAST	LUNCH	DINNER
OATMEAL Fresh fruit	PRESSURE-COOKED BROWN RICE LUSCIOUS LEEKS PINTO BEANS RUTABAGA PICKLES Fresh fruit	MISO SOUP BROILED WHITEFISH PRESSED CUCUMBER SALAD SAUTÉED GREENS (kale) BAKED SQUASH APPLE-LEMON KANTEN

* Tuesday *

BREAKFAST	LUNCH	DINNER
MILLET WITH VEGETABLES Fresh fruit	UDON NOODLES IN BROTH CHINESE-STYLE VEGETABLES Fresh fruit	Broiled skinless chicken BOILED BROWN RICE, served with SCALLION, RED PEPPER, AND SESAME-SEED CONDIMENT STEAMED GREENS (Brussels sprouts) BAKED SQUASH BLUEBERRY CRISP Beverage

* Wednesday *

BREAKFAST	LUNCH	DINNER
Stewed prunes, figs, and raisins	MACARONI AND BEAN SALAD CABBAGE WITH CUMIN	BAKED SALMON ROASTED POTATOES Salad with chickpeas, Bermuda onions, and broccoli, and MISO DRESSING APPLES WITH APRICOT SAUCE

* Thursday *

BREAKFAST	LUNCH	DINNER
QUINOA PORRIDGE Fresh fruit	BROILED WHITEFISH Salad with broccoli and cauliflower, and SESAME-LEMON DRESSING	BOILED BROWN RICE with SCALLION, RED PEPPER, AND SESAME-SEED CONDIMENT BAKED SQUASH SCRAMBLED TOFU CHINESE-STYLE VEGETABLES STEAMED GREENS (kale)

* Friday *

BREAKFAST	LUNCH	DINNER
Two-egg omelette with onions, mushrooms, tomatoes, and broccoli	Vegetable soup Salad with any three vegetables, and VINAIGRETTE DRESSING Fresh fruit	GREEN LENTIL SOUP WITH POTATO BUCKWHEAT AND BOWS DAIKON RADISH SALAD MARINATED VEGETABLES SAUTÉED GREENS (collards) BLUEBERRY CRISP

* Saturday *

BREAKFAST	LUNCH	DINNER
Stewed prunes, figs, and raisins	MACARONI AND BEAN SALAD CABBAGE WITH CUMIN	BAKED SALMON ROASTED POTATOES Salad with chickpeas, Bermuda onions, and broccoli, and MISO DRESSING APPLES WITH APRICOT SAUCE

WEEK THREE

* Sunday *

BREAKFAST	LUNCH	DINNER
OATMEAL	MACARONI AND BEAN SALAD STEAMED GREENS (watercress) Fresh fruit salad	MISO SOUP Broiled skinless chicken WILD RICE PILAF CABBAGE WITH CUMIN Salad with three vegetables, and TOFU DRESSING Roasted seeds and raisins

* Monday *

BREAKFAST	LUNCH	DINNER
STEWED PEACHES, blueberries, and raisins	COLD SOBA NOODLES WITH GINGER-SESAME SAUCE STEAMED GREENS (broccoli) Fresh fruit salad	BAKED SALMON CHINESE-STYLE VEGETABLES PLAIN BAKED POTATO Salad with three vegetables, and LEMON DRESSING Kuzu fruit dessert

* Tuesday *

BREAKFAST	LUNCH	DINNER
SCRAMBLED TOFU Fresh fruit	GREEN LENTIL SOUP WITH POTATO	Broiled skinless chicken ROOT STEW PRESSED CUCUMBER SALAD STEAMED GREENS (kale) BLUEBERRY CRISP

* Wednesday *

BREAKFAST	LUNCH	DINNER
Stewed prunes, figs, and raisins	BUCKWHEAT AND BOWS CABBAGE WITH CUMIN Fresh fruit salad	BROILED WHITEFISH ROASTED POTATOES RATATOUILLE Salad with broccoli, cauliflower, and carrots, and TOFU DRESSING Unsweetened applesauce

* Thursday *

BREAKFAST	LUNCH	DINNER
OATMEAL	MARINATED CHICKPEA SALAD WILD RICE PILAF STEAMED GREENS (watercress)	FRIED RICE WITH SHRIMP AND VEGETABLES BAKED SQUASH SAUTÉED GREENS (Brussels sprouts) DAIKON RADISH SALAD BLUEBERRY CRISP

* Friday *

BREAKFAST	LUNCH	DINNER
QUINOA PORRIDGE Fresh fruit	SHIITAKE AND BARLEY SOUP Salad with chickpeas and Bermuda onions, and SESAME-LEMON DRESSING	LINGUINI WITH WHITE CLAM SAUCE BOILED CARROTS AND PARSNIPS SAUTÉED GREENS (asparagus) APPLE-LEMON KANTEN

* Saturday *

BREAKFAST	LUNCH	DINNER
MILLET WITH VEGETABLES	BAKED SWEET POTATO OR YAM	MISO SOUP
	STEAMED GREENS (kale)	Broiled skinless chicken
	UDON NOODLES IN BROTH	Salad with three vegetables, and VINAIGRETTE DRESSING
		ROASTED POTATOES
		RUTABAGA PICKLES
		BLUEBERRY CRISP

The next chapter contains the recipes needed to prepare these meals. They are easy to follow and easy to prepare.

14

Recipes and Food Preparation Tips

IN THIS CHAPTER THERE ARE MORE THAN 50 recipes for Phase 1 and Phase 2 dishes. In Phase 1, the cooking tends to be light and shorter in duration than for the Phase 2 foods. The exceptions are the beans and the larger, thicker vegetables such as potatoes and squash.

Utensils

Whole foods cooking is, in many ways, a lot easier and cleaner than cooking meat, chicken, and fatty foods. For one thing, the most common cooking ingredient is water. We don't use lard, or fat, and we minimize oil in cooking. Still, learning to cook vegetables, beans, and grains so that they are delicious and satisfying does take some time, trial and error, and a little study. It also takes the right cooking utensils. Here's a short list of utensils and some advice to help you get started.

Pots

Avoid aluminum pots. Aluminum chips and molecules from the pot leach into food. There is still some concern over the possible neurological effects of aluminum. Instead, use stainless-steel, cast-iron, glass, porcelain, stoneware, and nonstick-coated pans and bakeware.

Buy a good pressure cooker. This is an old-fashioned pot that was once a fixture in every American kitchen. Today, people don't do much cooking, and some who do cook worry about possible accidents with pressure cookers. The pots made today are safe, highly convenient, and make it easier to prepare delicious food. Read the instructions when you purchase your pressure cooker; keep the pot top, regulator, and gasket clean, and you won't have any trouble with your pressure cooker. Use it regularly, and you'll be glad you have it. Pressure cooking locks in the flavor of foods, especially whole grains, making the grains sweet, nutty-flavored, and delicious. You can combine whole grains and beans to make a luscious dish. You can also pressure-cook beans and thick vegetable combinations. Peel and chop a winter squash into two-inch chunks; cut up two carrots into coins, and slice an onion into quarters. Pressure-cook them all together in a half-inch of water for 10 minutes to make a soft, sweet, delicious vegetable medley. You can add other root vegetables, such as parsnips and burdock, as well as beans to the mix to create rich and exotic entrées.

Vegetable Knife

Shop around for a knife that feels good in your hand and that can hold a sharp edge. Many people like a 7-inch knife, with a rectangular, 1½-inch wide stainless-steel blade. The rectangular blade is perfect for cutting vegetables, because it provides a nice balance and leverage for downward chopping.

Grater

Buy a stainless-steel or porcelain vegetable grater. You'll want a good grater to add freshly grated ginger, garlic, and other condiments to your food. You can also grate carrots for salad, and combine grated carrots and daikon radish to make a pleasing, slightly pungent, palate-clearing condiment to accompany a salad.

Steamer Basket

As you will see from the recipes that follow, I like steaming vegetables. It's a quick and nutrient-sparing way of preparing vegetables. You can steam most greens and leafy vegetables in 5 to 7 minutes. Carrots, parsnips, turnips, rutabagas, and other roots can also be steamed. Steaming is a light form of cooking that prevents the loss of nutrients, while allowing the natural flavors and colors of plant foods to be retained. You can buy a stainless-steel or a bamboo steamer. In no time, you'll wonder how you got along without one.

Wooden Spoons

Wooden spoons of various lengths are essential for mixing and preparing vegetables and grains while they're cooking.

Food Preparation Tips

There are myriad ways to make both the Phase 1 and 2 diets easy to follow, especially on days when you are pressed for time. Here are some ideas to cut preparation time:

- Cook beans, soups, and other time-consuming entrées on, say, Wednesday night and the weekends. Refrigerate and just reheat when you get home from work. You can also freeze portions and defrost and reheat as needed.
- Soak dried beans, peas, lentils, and chickpeas overnight or during the day. Discard the soaking water to make the beans easier to digest.
- Buy jarred beans. Most supermarkets today have jarred beans, such as black beans, chickpeas, and pinto beans, many organically grown. All you have to do is open the jar, slice up some carrots, red or green peppers, and onions and cook them together in a sauce pan. Add some spices, such as cayenne pepper, and you've got a delicious meal in less than 15 minutes.
- Buy plenty of jarred, canned, and dehydrated soups. Be sure that the soups do not include oil, and try to purchase only the highest quality. There are many high-quality soups available that only need to be heated, or prepared by adding water. Throughout the menus I refer to such soups

as vegetable soup. You can buy all types of soups, including split pea, lentil, lima bean, and other vegetable-based soups.

* Pressure-cook large vegetables such as squash to shorten cooking time. Chop up the squash in chunks, place in a pressure cooker, add water, and bring to pressure. That will require about 10 minutes; cook for another 10 minutes and you've got a delicious entrée. Place the squash in a blender or food processor; add other cooked vegetables such as carrots, scallions, or some herbs; blend, reheat, and serve as a delicious squash soup (see recipes in the recipe section).

* Try exotic ready-made foods that are rich in protein and low in fat. Among these are seitan (pronounced "say-tan"), which is wheat gluten. Seitan has a very hearty, meaty consistency and is a great meat substitute. It's rich in protein and delicious in soups and stews. It requires no real cooking time; just chop it up and add it to soup and heat. It's ready when the soup is hot. Another easy-to-prepare food that's delicious and great for your health is tempeh (see also chapter 9), a whole-soybean patty that's rich in protein, minerals, vitamins, and isoflavones. You can boil it in water for 15 minutes; add vegetables and you've got a great high-protein entrée.

* Use leftovers creatively. Make more than you need for dinner and you've got your lunch already taken care of.

* When you're on the Phase 2 diet, use high-quality noodles such as whole-wheat noodles, semolina, Italian noodles, Japanese udon (a wide, sifted wheat noodle), Japanese soba (a buckwheat noodle), and ramen packages. Noodles, as you know, are quick-cooking. Add vegetables to the broth and some shoyu or miso; both are high-quality soup and sauce bases made from fermented soybeans (see chapter 9 for more on miso and shoyu). Noodle soup that includes a variety of vegetables can be a complete meal in a single pot.

No doubt you will come up with a lot of your own ideas for making this program work for you.

To beef up the anti-inflammatory value of each meal, include anti-inflammatory garnishes such as flaxseeds. These can be added to fruit, vegetable, or grain dishes.

Also, there are lots of healthful condiments that can be added to your meals to give them more zest and flavor. Here are some of the condiments that I recommend.

* Balsamic vinegar
* Brown-rice vinegar
* Wine vinegars
* Fresh grated ginger root
* Horseradish
* Lemon and lemon juice
* Mustard
* Black and cayenne pepper
* Low-sodium sauerkraut
* Salsa
* Sea salt
* Salt substitute
* Miso
* Allium-rich vegetables such as garlic, onions, and scallions (very anti-inflammatory)

Bon appétit!

Phase 1 Recipes

VEGETABLES

Boiled Carrots and Parsnips

1 pound carrots, thinly sliced
1 pound parsnips, thinly sliced
½ cup water

✳ Place the carrots and parsnips in a saucepan and cover with water. Cover and boil for 10 minutes.

MAKES 4 SERVINGS

Chinese-Style Vegetables

1 large onion, sliced
4 cups sliced cabbage
1 large carrot, diced
1 clove garlic, grated
2 cups water
1 cup snow peas
2 scallions, chopped
1 teaspoon brown-rice or red wine vinegar
1 tablespoon shoyu
1 teaspoon grated ginger
1 tablespoon kuzu diluted in 1 cup water (optional)
1 teaspoon ground and roasted flaxseeds (optional)

✳ Place onion, carrot, and cabbage in a large skillet. Add garlic and two cups of water and simmer, covered, for 3 to 5 minutes. Add snow peas and scallions and simmer 2 minutes longer. Add vinegar, shoyu, ginger, and kuzu (if desired) and stir until thick. Sprinkle roasted flaxseeds over vegetables, if desired.

MAKES 3 SERVINGS

Luscious Leeks

5 to 6 leeks, sliced lengthwise
1 tablespoon olive oil
1 teaspoon shoyu sauce
3 teaspoons prepared mustard
2 teaspoons brown-rice syrup
1 teaspoon balsamic vinegar

✳ Wash leeks carefully and sauté, covered, in olive oil for about 25 minutes. Occasionally lift cover and stir vegetables. Remove cover and continue cooking until there is no remaining liquid. Remove from heat. Put shoyu, brown-rice syrup, mustard, and vinegar in a covered jar and shake. Add to the leeks and serve over any grain dish.

MAKES 3 SERVINGS

Steamed Greens

❋ Thoroughly rinse 4 cups green vegetables. Choose from or mix together asparagus, broccoli, Brussels sprouts, kale, mustard greens, watercress, collard greens, bok choy, or any other dark-green vegetable. Cut into bite-size pieces.

❋ Put approximately ½ inch of water in the bottom of a small skillet. You can use a steamer basket or put the vegetables directly into the water.

❋ Place sliced greens in water and cover. Steam for 3 to 7 minutes, until greens are soft but still retain their color.

MAKES 2 SERVINGS

Water-Sautéed Carrots, Onions, and Summer Squash

4 onions, diced

4 large carrots, diced

⅛ cup water

2 large summer squash, diced

1 tablespoon shoyu

❋ Place ¼ inch of water in the bottom of a small skillet, then add onions and carrots. Cook, covered, for 5 minutes. Add summer squash and shoyu, and cook, covered, 5 minutes more.

MAKES 3 SERVINGS

CRUCIFEROUS AND ROOT VEGETABLES

Baked Squash

1 medium acorn or butternut squash, cut in half

❋ Preheat oven to 450 degrees. Scoop out the seeds from the squash and discard. Place squash skin side up in a baking dish. Cook for 1 hour or until it can easily be pierced with a fork.

MAKES 4 SERVINGS

Baked Sweet Potato or Baked Yam

1 sweet potato or yam

✳ Preheat oven to 400 degrees. Wrap sweet potato or yam in foil. Bake for 2 hours, or until fork can easily be inserted.

MAKES 2 SERVINGS

Cabbage with Cumin

2 tablespoons olive oil
1 head cabbage, finely chopped
1 tablespoon sea salt
1 tablespoon cumin powder
1⅛ cups water (optional)

✳ Sauté all ingredients together for 5 minutes, adding water if necessary. Then cover and steam for an additional 5 minutes.

MAKES 4 SERVINGS

Daikon Radish Salad

1 cup grated daikon radish
1 cup grated carrot
½ teaspoon salt
Juice of 1 lemon
½ cup thinly sliced scallions

✳ Mix together and serve.

MAKES 3 SERVINGS

Daikon Radish with Shoyu

1 daikon radish, sliced
1 tablespoon shoyu

❋ Place daikon and shoyu in a small pot with water to cover. Boil until fork can be easily inserted into the daikon, about 15 minutes.

MAKES 1 SERVING

Plain Baked Potato

1 baking potato

❋ Preheat oven to 350 degrees. Scrub potato clean. Wrap in foil and bake 1½ to 2 hours. Flavor with chives, scallions, salsa, or other condiments suggested on page 223.

MAKES 1 SERVING

Root Stew

1 onion, chopped
1 sweet potato, cubed
4 medium carrots, sliced
1 parsnip, sliced
1 small winter squash, sliced
½ cup water
½ teaspoon salt

❋ Layer vegetables in a cast-iron or stainless-steel pot with cover and add water and salt. Bring to a boil, turn down, and cook, covered, on very low heat for at least an hour, until vegetables are very soft.

MAKES 4 SERVINGS

Rutabaga Pickle

2 cups rutabaga, finely chopped
Shoyu
Water

✳ Place rutabaga in pickle press, small ceramic crock, or bowl. Prepare a mixture of half water and half shoyu to cover the rutabaga. Put top on pickle press or some kind of weight on vegetables in the crock or bowl. Press rutabaga for 4 hours or overnight.

MAKES 4 SERVINGS

BEANS AND PULSES (DRIED PEAS)

Adzuki Beans

2 cups adzuki beans, washed and presoaked
8 cups water
3 tablespoons barley miso
3 tablespoons apple butter

✳ Soak beans for 6 hours or overnight. Discard soaking water. When ready to cook the beans, place them in 8 cups of water and bring to boil. Reduce heat and simmer covered for 1½ hours or until beans are soft. Combine miso with apple butter and add to beans. Simmer together for 10 minutes, or until most of the liquid is absorbed. Remove from heat and serve.

MAKES 2 SERVINGS

Boiled Beans

Kidney beans, pinto beans, black beans, or adzuki beans

✳ Wash beans and pick over for stones. Soak 1 cup of beans overnight in 5 cups water. Discard the soaking water. Place in pot with 3 cups of water and bring to a boil, being careful not to let the beans boil over. Boil briskly, uncovered, until the beans are soft, 1½ to 2 hours.

✳ When beans are soft, remove from heat; add salt, shoyu, or miso; and serve.

✳ To pressure-cook beans (which can be far easier than boiling them): Wash and pick over beans for stones. Be sure the pressure cooker regulator is clear and clean before pressure-cooking beans, because beans can clog a regulator that is already dirty and cause accidents during cooking.

✳ Place in the pot 3 cups of water per 1 cup of beans. Put on the pressure-cooker cover and lock shut. Bring to pressure, as indicated by the hissing of the regulator; this usually takes approximately 10 minutes. Reduce heat to low and cook for 45 minutes. Run pot under cold water before removing the lid.

MAKES 2 SERVINGS

Green Lentil Soup with Potato

This recipe can be further enhanced by adding some seitan (see p. 222). Seitan is made from wheat gluten. It is very hearty, chewy, and delicious. It can be purchased in most natural-foods stores.

7 cups water
1 cup green lentils
*   (lentils do not need presoaking)*
1 small onion, diced
2 carrots, diced
2 stalks celery, diced
6 small potatoes, cut in quarters
1 clove garlic, grated
1 cup seitan (optional)
Shoyu (to taste)
1 scallion, chopped (garnish)

✳ Boil lentils in 7 cups water until soft. Cut vegetables and add to the lentils, along with potato and garlic. (Add seitan at this point, if desired.)

Cook on medium heat, covered, for 30 minutes. Add shoyu to taste and simmer for 10 minutes longer. Garnish with scallion.

MAKES 3 SERVINGS

Marinated Chickpea Salad

> 3 cups cooked chickpeas (canned or jarred is fine)
> 2 tablespoons olive oil
> 3 tablespoons vinegar
> Pinch of sea salt
> 6 red radishes, diced
> 1 small cucumber, peeled and diced
> 2 stalks celery, diced
> ½ cup finely chopped watercress
> 1 tablespoon chopped fresh parsley
> 1 teaspoon fresh dill

✳ Marinate the chickpeas in oil, vinegar, and sea salt. Combine with vegetables and add fresh parsley and dill.

MAKES 3 SERVINGS

Pinto Beans

> 2 cups presoaked pinto beans
> 10 cups water
> 1 onion, diced
> 1 green pepper, diced
> 1 teaspoon grated garlic
> 1 teaspoon cumin
> 1 teaspoon cayenne pepper
> Shoyu, miso, or salt (to taste)

✳ Cook pinto beans in a large pot with water for 2 hours. Drain the beans. Sauté onion, green pepper, garlic, cumin, cayenne, and shoyu, miso, or salt to taste. Add the beans and continue to sauté for 10 minutes, covered.

✳ You can use canned beans in this recipe if you are in a hurry.

Scrambled Tofu

1 onion, diced
1 carrot, diced
½ rib celery, diced
1 cake soft tofu
1 teaspoon cumin
1 teaspoon turmeric
¼ teaspoon black pepper

✳ Steam onion, carrot, and celery in water for 3 minutes. Crumble up the tofu and add to the mixture. Add cumin, pepper, and turmeric. Cook covered for 10 minutes.

MAKES 2 SERVINGS

SOUPS

Miso Soup

1 onion, diced
1 carrot, diced
½ cabbage, diced
4 shiitake mushrooms, soaked, sliced, and tips of stems removed
5 cups water
3 tablespoons miso
1 scallion, sliced (garnish)
1 teaspoon grated ginger (garnish)

✳ Place onion, carrot, cabbage, and mushrooms in a pot with 5 cups water. Bring to a boil. Reduce to low flame, cover, and simmer 20 minutes.

Dissolve miso in a cup of the broth and return to the soup. Simmer 10 minutes longer. Remove from heat and serve garnished with scallions and grated ginger.

MAKES 3 SERVINGS

Red Lentil Soup

1 cup red lentils
6 bay leaves
1 large onion, cut into ½-inch pieces
2 medium carrots, cut into ½-inch pieces
2 beets, cut into ½-inch pieces
¼ cup miso
Handful of chopped parsley (garnish)

✳ Wash and drain the lentils and cook them for 40 minutes with the bay leaves. Remove bay leaves. Add the vegetables to lentils and cook for 1 hour. Puree or blend well. Dissolve miso in a little water and add. Heat pureed mixture on low for 10 minutes. Sprinkle with parsley and serve.

MAKES 3 SERVINGS

Shiitake and Barley Soup

½ cup pearled barley
10 shiitake mushrooms, whole
1 onion, chopped
2 carrots, sliced
7 leaves Chinese cabbage, chopped
½ cup miso
1 scallion, sliced (garnish)
1 teaspoon grated ginger (garnish)

✳ Fill a pot with water. Add shiitake mushrooms and pearled barley. Bring to a boil. Turn down flame and simmer for 20 minutes. Take out mushrooms with a spatula, dice them, and return them to broth. Add the onion, carrots, and Chinese cabbage leaves to soup. Cover and simmer for at least 1 hour. Ladle out some broth and mix miso into it. Return to pot and simmer on low for 20 minutes, but do not allow to boil. Garnish with scallion and grated ginger.

MAKES 4 SERVINGS

Squash Soup

8 cups seeded and cubed winter squash (butternut or acorn)
1 cup water
1 large sweet potato
10 tablespoons miso (or to taste)

✳ Place squash in a pressure cooker with sweet potato and 1 cup of water. Bring to pressure and cook on low for 10 minutes. Cool down cooker before opening. Puree vegetables in a blender or food processor. Transfer to pot and reheat. Add miso and more water if you would like a more liquid consistency. Cook on low for 10 minutes.

MAKES 3 SERVINGS

DRESSINGS

Lemon Dressing

Juice of 3 lemons
½ cup shoyu

✳ Mix together and serve.
MAKES 2 SERVINGS

Orange Dressing

3 tablespoons white miso
½ cup orange juice

✳ Blend thoroughly.
MAKES 2 SERVINGS

Scallion, Red Pepper, and Sesame-Seed Condiment

6 scallions, thinly sliced
1 red pepper, diced
1 tablespoon miso
2 tablespoons roasted sesame seeds

✳ Place scallions and red pepper in a pot with a little water and steam for 5 minutes. Add miso, stir, and cook on low flame for 5 minutes more. Blend in roasted sesame seeds.

MAKES 3 SERVINGS

Tofu Dressing

½ teaspoon grated ginger
1 cake soft tofu
¼ cup water
2 tablespoons white miso
2 tablespoons vinegar

✳ Blend all ingredients until creamy.

MAKES 2 SERVINGS

FRUIT DESSERTS

Apple-Lemon Kanten

10 cups apple juice
4 cups water
⅛ teaspoon salt
7 tablespoons agar-agar flakes
6 medium apples, cored and sliced
1 tablespoon grated lemon rind
Juice of 1 medium lemon

✳ Place apple juice and water in a saucepan and heat. When the liquid comes to a boil, reduce heat and add salt and agar-agar, stirring constantly. Stir in apples, lemon rind, and lemon juice. Simmer for 15 minutes, pour into a dish, and allow to chill in the refrigerator until it sets.

MAKES 4 SERVINGS

Stewed Peaches

4 pounds fresh peaches
Water to cover
2 teaspoons vanilla
Grated rind of 1 lemon

✳ Wash peaches and halve them lengthwise, separating pulp from pit. Cut each half into three slices. Place peaches in a saucepan, cover with water, and add vanilla and lemon rind. Bring to a boil, lower heat, and simmer, covered, for 5 minutes. Serve at room temperature or cool.

MAKES 5 SERVINGS

Phase 2 Recipes

After you achieve the Phase 1 goals, you will go on to Phase 2, but all the foods that you can eat during Phase 1 should also be eaten on Phase 2. Don't stop eating steamed vegetables just because you can add a small amount of olive oil on Phase 2. Steaming, boiling, and baking vegetables are the preferred ways of preparing them. These cooking methods can ensure your long-term good health.

VEGETABLES

Marinated Vegetables

⅔ cup olive oil
1 lemon juice
2 teaspoons sea salt

5 cups coarsely chopped vegetables (broccoli, cauliflower, Brussels
sprouts, zucchini, carrot, and/or green beans)

❋ Blend olive oil, lemon juice, and salt to make a marinade. Toss with
cut-up vegetables. Marinate in refrigerator for 24 hours, stir, and serve.

MAKES 4 SERVINGS

Pressed Cucumber Salad

4 cucumbers, peeled and sliced
1 teaspoon sea salt
1 teaspoon shoyu
1 teaspoon toasted sesame oil
1 teaspoon brown-rice vinegar
3 tablespoons toasted sesame seeds (garnish)

❋ Place sliced cucumber and sea salt in a pickle press or in a bowl with a
weight on top of the cucumbers. Press for an hour or more and drain off the
liquid. Rinse off the salt. Add mixture of shoyu, sesame oil, and brown-rice
vinegar to the cucumbers and garnish with toasted sesame seeds.

MAKES 4 SERVINGS

Ratatouille

1 onion, diced
3 large yellow summer squashes, sliced
2 tomatoes, diced
Pinch of salt

❋ Place all ingredients in a pot with a little bit of water and steam a few
minutes until vegetables are soft.

MAKES 2 SERVINGS

Roasted Potatoes

1 pound small potatoes (yellow or red)
1 tablespoon olive oil
Salt and pepper (to taste)

✳ Preheat oven to 350 degrees. Scrub and dry the potatoes. Coat them lightly with oil and season with salt and pepper. Place in an oven pan and roast for 1½ hours or until a fork can be inserted easily into each potato.

MAKES 2 SERVINGS

Sautéed Carrots, Onions, and Summer Squash

1 tablespoon olive oil
4 onions, diced
4 large carrots, diced
2 large summer squash (yellow or zucchini), diced
1 tablespoon shoyu

✳ Heat oil in skillet and add onions and carrots. Cook, covered, for 5 minutes. Add the summer squash and shoyu and cook, covered, 5 minutes more.

MAKES 3 SERVINGS

Sautéed Greens

2 tablespoons olive oil
1 teaspoon shoyu
1 clove garlic, crushed
2 cups sliced green vegetables (asparagus, broccoli, Brussels sprouts, collard greens, kale, mustard greens, watercress, or any other dark-green vegetable)

✳ Place oil, shoyu, garlic, and greens in a skillet. Sauté for 2 to 5 minutes. Green are done when they are soft but still retain their color.

MAKES 2 SERVINGS

Boiled Brown Rice

1 cup brown rice, washed
2 cups water
Pinch of sea salt

✳ Place rice, water, and salt in a stainless-steel pot and bring to a boil. Turn heat down to low and cover. Simmer for 1 hour or a little longer if the rice is too watery.

MAKES 2 SERVINGS

Buckwheat and Bows

8 cups water
1 teaspoon sea salt
2 cups roasted buckwheat groats (you can buy them already roasted)
1 onion, minced
½ pound bowtie noodles, already cooked
1 teaspoon prepared mustard
1 teaspoon shoyu
½ cup minced parsley (garnish)

✳ Bring the water and salt to a boil. Add buckwheat and onion and cook for 20 minutes, until water has been absorbed. Mix in noodles, mustard, and shoyu. Garnish with parsley.

MAKES 3 SERVINGS

Fried Rice with Shrimp and Vegetables

1 tablespoon olive oil
1 clove garlic, minced
1 cup broccoli florets
1 cup thinly sliced carrots
1 cup cooked rice

1 cup thinly sliced scallions

¼ pound cooked shrimp

1 tablespoon shoyu

¼ teaspoon vinegar

1 teaspoon grated ginger

✳ Heat oil in a skillet. Add garlic, broccoli, and carrots and stir for 10 seconds. Cover and cook a few minutes longer until broccoli is tender. Add the cooked rice, scallions, shrimp, shoyu, vinegar, and ginger. Stir together until everything is well mixed and rice is coated with the sauce.

MAKES 3 SERVINGS

Millet with Vegetables

6 cups water

1 cup millet, washed

1 onion, diced

1 carrot, diced

½ head cauliflower, separated into small florets

1 clove garlic, minced

½ teaspoon sea salt

✳ Place all ingredients in a pot and bring to boil. Lower heat and cook, covered, for 45 minutes. If there is still a lot of unabsorbed water left in the millet when you turn the flame off, allow the dish to sit covered for a while, as the millet will absorb it.

MAKES 3 SERVINGS

Oatmeal

1 cup steel-cut oats, washed

2 cups water

Handful of raisins

Pinch of sea salt

1 tablespoon roasted flaxseeds (garnish)

✳ Place oats, water, raisins, and salt in a pot and boil, covered, for 15 minutes. Garnish with roasted flaxseeds.

MAKES 2 SERVINGS

Pressure-cooked Brown Rice

1 cup brown rice, washed
½ cup water
Pinch of sea salt

✳ Place rice, water, and salt in a pressure cooker and bring to pressure. As soon as pressure gauge begins to jiggle and hiss, reduce heat to low and cook for 45 minutes. Remove from heat and allow to cool. Do not attempt to open the pressure cooker until it has cooled off.

MAKES 3 SERVINGS

Quinoa Porridge

1 cup water
1 cup rinsed quinoa
½ cup grated or chopped carrots
Pinch of sea salt
1 tablespoon toasted flaxseeds
brown-rice syrup, to taste (optional)

✳ Place water, quinoa, carrots, and salt in a medium saucepan. Bring to a boil, cover, and cook on low for 15 minutes. Add flaxseeds and sweetener, such as brown-rice syrup, if desired.

MAKES 2 SERVINGS

Wild Rice Pilaf

1 onion, chopped
1 tablespoon olive oil
3 cups water
3 tablespoons shoyu

1¾ cups long-grain brown rice
¼ cup wild rice

✳ In a medium-sized skillet, sauté onion in oil. In a pot bring water and
shoyu to a boil. Add rice and onion to water, cover, and cook over low heat
for 1 hour.

MAKES 3 SERVINGS

NOODLES AND PASTA

Cold Soba Noodles with Ginger-Sesame Sauce

½ pound soba noodles
6 cups water
½ teaspoon sea salt
¼ cup shoyu
2 tablespoons unrefined sesame oil
1 tablespoon roasted sesame oil
1 tablespoon brown-rice vinegar
2 teaspoons maple syrup
1 teaspoon grated ginger
1 teaspoon minced garlic
1 cup chopped scallions
2 tablespoons roughly ground, toasted sesame seeds

✳ Boil soba noodles in lightly salted water until soft. Drain and rinse well
with cool water. Drain again. Whisk together shoyu, sesame oils, maple
syrup, ginger, and garlic. Pour dressing over cooked noodles and mix in
scallions and sesame seeds.

MAKES 2 SERVINGS

Linguini with White Clam Sauce

10 cups water
Pinch sea salt

1 pound linguini

1 tablespoon olive oil

2 cloves garlic, minced

4 scallions, minced

⅔ cup minced parsley

15 button mushrooms, sliced into small pieces

1 16-ounce can of clams

2 tablespoons shoyu

✳ Boil water, add salt and linguini, and cook for 10 minutes or until linguine is al dente. Drain and rinse briefly with cold water. Sauté vegetables in olive oil in a skillet. Cover and simmer for 5 minutes. Add the canned clams along with the juice and the shoyu. Serve over cooked noodles.

MAKES 3 SERVINGS

Macaroni and Bean Salad

3 cups cooked whole-wheat macaroni

1½ cups cooked kidney beans

4 scallions, finely chopped

2 celery stalks, finely chopped

Handful of finely chopped parsley

Mustard Dressing (recipe below)

✳ In a large bowl, combine the macaroni and beans (canned or jarred beans may be used). Add the chopped scallions, celery, and parsley to the macaroni mixture. Toss with Mustard Dressing and allow to stand for 15 minutes before serving.

MAKES 3 SERVINGS

Mustard Dressing

6 tablespoons lemon juice

4 tablespoons shoyu

2 teaspoons mustard

2 tablespoons sesame tahini
6 tablespoons water

✳ Place the ingredients in a small jar, cover, and shake thoroughly until well blended.

MAKES 3 SERVINGS

Udon Noodles in Broth

6 cups water
1 package (½ pound) udon noodles
4 shiitake mushrooms, soaked, sliced, and stems removed
½ cake firm tofu, cubed
6 broccoli florets
Shoyu (to taste)
Chopped scallions (garnish)

✳ Bring water to a boil. Add noodles and cook until soft. Remove noodles, but retain the noodle water. Rinse noodles under cold water, and drain. Place shiitake mushrooms and tofu in noodle water and cook for 10 minutes. Add broccoli and cook for 5 more minutes or until broccoli is soft but still bright green. Turn off flame and allow to cool in the refrigerator. When the broth is cool, add shoyu to taste, put the noodles in individual bowls, and add broth and vegetables over each serving. Sprinkle with chopped scallions.

MAKES 2 SERVINGS

FISH

Baked Salmon

3 tablespoons olive oil
1 teaspoon Worcestershire sauce
1 onion, minced
2 pounds salmon fillet

❋ Preheat oven to 350 degrees. In a bowl, combine oil, Worcestershire sauce, and minced onion. Place salmon in shallow baking dish, cover with sauce, and bake for about 30 minutes.

MAKES 4 SERVINGS

Broiled Whitefish

2 *pounds whitefish*
2 *tablespoons shoyu*
2 *tablespoons sesame oil*
Juice of 1 lemon

❋ Place fish on baking dish and sprinkle with shoyu, lemon juice, and sesame oil. Broil until fish flakes easily.

MAKES 4 SERVINGS

DRESSINGS AND SAUCES

Miso Dressing

3 *tablespoons white miso*
1 *tablespoon brown-rice vinegar*
1 *teaspoon toasted sesame oil*
1 *clove garlic, grated*
1 *teaspoon grated ginger*

❋ Blend all ingredients thoroughly.

MAKES 2 SERVINGS

Sesame-Lemon Dressing

2 *tablespoons sesame oil*
2 *tablespoons lemon juice*
1 *tablespoon brown-rice vinegar*

2 tablespoons shoyu

½ cup water

✳ Put all ingredients in a covered jar and shake until well mixed.

MAKES 2 SERVINGS

Vinaigrette Dressing

2 tablespoons minced onion

1 tablespoon prepared mustard

3 tablespoons brown-rice vinegar

½ tablespoon olive oil

1 teaspoon shoyu

✳ Put all ingredients in a covered jar and shake until well mixed.

MAKES 2 SERVINGS

FRUIT DESSERTS

Apples with Apricot Sauce

½ pound dried apricots

Pinch sea salt

8 apples, washed, cored, and cut into small pieces

Handful toasted walnuts (garnish)

✳ Place apricots in a bowl and cover them with water. Soak for an hour. Place apricots and the water in a saucepan and add salt. Bring to a boil, and simmer for 15 minutes, until soft. Place the apples in another pot in ½ inch of water and simmer for about 10 minutes. Mash the apricots in a separate bowl and mix with the juice from the apples to make a sauce. If the sauce is too thick, add a little water. Dish out some of the apples, cover with the sauce, and garnish with walnuts.

MAKES 4 SERVINGS

Blueberry Crisp

> 4 cups blueberries
> 1 cup apple juice
> 2 tablespoons brown-rice syrup
> 2 tablespoons kuzu (dissolved in 5 tablespoons water)
> 3 cups rolled oats
> Pinch sea salt
> 3 tablespoons maple syrup

✳ Preheat oven to 350 degrees. Place blueberries, apple juice, and brown-rice syrup in a pot and simmer. Add dissolved kuzu and stir until mixture is thickened. In a mixing bowl combine oats, salt, and maple syrup. Place blueberry mixture in a baking dish and cover with the oats mixture. Bake for 30 minutes.

MAKES 4 SERVINGS

Index of Recipes

References

Chapter 1: A New Understanding of Heart Disease

Abbasi, F., B. W. Brown Jr., C. Lamendola, et al. 2002. Relationship between obesity, insulin resistance, and coronary heart disease risk. *J. Am. Coll. Cardiol.* 40:937–43.

Almagor, M., A. Keren, and S. Banai. 2003. Increased C-reactive protein level after coronary stent implantation in patients with stable coronary artery disease. *Am. Heart J.* 145:248–53.

Chung B. H., F. Franklin, B. H. Cho, et al. 1998. Potencies of lipoproteins in fasting and postprandial plasma to accept additional cholesterol molecules released from cell membranes. *Arterioscler. Thromb. Vasc. Biol.* 18:1217–30.

Cnop, M., P. J. Havel, K. M. Utzschneider, et al. 2003 (in print). Relationship of adiponectin to body fat distribution, insulin sensitivity and plasma lipoproteins: evidence for independent roles of age and sex. *Diabetologia* 10.

Das, U. N. 2001. Is obesity an inflammatory condition? *Nutrition* 17:953–66.

Djaldetti, M., H. Salman, M. Bergman, et al. 2002. Phagocytosis—the mighty weapon of the silent warriors. *Microsc. Res. Tech.* 57:421–31.

Fleming, R. M. 2003. Caloric intake, not carbohydrate or fat consumption, determines weight loss. *Am. J. Med.* 114:78.

——. 2000a. The clinical importance of risk factor modification: looking at both myocardial viability (MV) and myocardial perfusion imaging (MPI). *International J. Angiol.* 9:55–69.

——. 2000b. The natural progression of atherosclerosis in an untreated patient with hyperlipidemia: assessment via cardiac PET. *Intern. J. Angiol.* 9:70–73.

——. 1999. The pathogenesis of vascular disease. In *Textbook of Angiology*, ed. John C. Chang, pp. 787–98. New York: Springer-Verlag.

Fleming, R. M., L. Boyd, and M. Forster. 2000. Reversing heart disease in the new millennium—the Fleming Unified Theory. *Angiology* 51:617–29.

Fleming, R. M., K. Ketchum, D. M. Fleming, et al. 1996. Assessing the independent effect of dietary counseling and hypolipidemic medications on serum lipids. *Angiology* 47:831–40.

——. 1995. Treating hyperlipidemia in the elderly. *Angiology* 46:1075–83.

Harvard Women's Health Watch. February 2003. Your heart attack risk: inflammation counts.

Haszon I., F. Papp, J. Kovacs, et al. 2003 (in print). Platelet aggregation, blood viscosity and serum lipids in hypertensive and obese children. *Eur. J. Pediatr.* 4.

Lehr, H. A., T. A. Sagban, and C. J. Kirkpatrick. 2002. Atherosclerosis—progression by nonspecific activation of the immune system. *Med. Klin.* 97:229–35.

Magadle, R., P. Weiner, M. Beckerman, et al. 2002. C-reactive protein as a marker for active coronary artery disease in patients with chest pain in the emergency room. *Clin. Cardiol.* 25:456–60.

Muscari, A., L. Bastagli, G. Poggiopollini, et al. 2002. Different associations of C-reactive protein, fibrinogen and C3 with traditional risk factors in middle-aged men. *International J. Cardiol.* 83:63–71.

Pellaton, C., S. Kubli, F. Feihl, et al. 2002. Blunted vasodilatory responses in the cutaneous microcirculation of cigarette smokers. *Am. Heart. J.* 144: 268–74.

Reaven, G., and P. S. Tsao. 2003. Insulin resistance and compensatory hyperinsulinemia: the key player between cigarette smoking and cardiovascular disease? *J. Am. Coll. Cardiol.* 41:1044–47.

Ridker, P. M., N. Rifai, L. Rose, et al. 2002. Comparison of C-reactive protein and low-density lipoprotein cholesterol levels in the prediction of first cardiovascular events. *New Engl. J. Med.* 347:1557–65.

Superko, H. R., and N. A. Chronos. 2003. Hypercholesterolemia and dyslipidemia: issues for the clinician. *Curr. Treat. Options Cardiovasc. Med.* 5:35–50.

Vogel, R. A. 2002. Alcohol, heart disease, and mortality: a review. *Rev. Cardiovasc. Med.* 3:7–13.

Woodward, M., J. Oliphant, G. Lowe, et al. 2003. Contribution of contemporaneous risk factors to social inequality in coronary heart disease and all cause mortality. *Prev. Med.* 36:561–68.

Zavaroni, I., D. Ardigo, P. Massironi, et al. 2002. Do coronary heart disease risk factors change over time? *Metabolism* 51:1022–26.

Chapter 2: Cholesterol and Triglycerides

Ait-yhia, D., S. Madani, J. L. Savelli, et al. 2003. Dietary fish lowers blood pressure and alters tissue polyunsaturated fatty acid composition in spontaneously hypertensive rats. *Nutrition* 19:342–46.

Anderson, J. T., et al. 1962. Effect of dietary cholesterol on serum cholesterol levels in man? *Proceedings* 21:100.

Arnett, E. N., J. M. Isner, and D. R. Redwood. 1979. Coronary artery narrowing in coronary heart disease: comparison of cineangiographic and necropsy findings. *Ann. Intern. Med.* 91:350–56.

Calder, P. C. 2002. Dietary modification of inflammation with lipids. *Proc. Nutr. Soc.* 61:345–58.

Chenevard, R., D. Hurlimann, M. Bechir, et al. 2003. Selective COX-2 inhibition improves endothelial function in coronary artery disease. *Circulation* 107:405–9.

Christensen, B., A. Mosdol, L. Retterstol, et al. 2001. Abstention from filtered coffee reduces the concentrations of plasma homocysteine and serum cholesterol—a randomized controlled trial. *Am. J. Clin. Nutr.* 74:302–7.

Cicha, I., Y. Suzuki, N. Tateishi, et al. 2001. Enhancement of red blood cell aggregation by plasma triglycerides. *Clin. Hemorheol. Microcirc.* 24: 247–55.

Connor, W. E., M. T. Cerqueira, R. W. Connor, et al. 1978. The plasma lipids, lipoproteins, and diet of the Tarahumara Indians of Mexico. *Am. J. Clin. Nutr.* 31:1131–42.

Duvernoy, C. S., and L. Mosca. 1999. Coronary heart disease in women: why the differences matter; they can affect diagnosis, treatment, outcomes, and preventive efforts. *J. Crit. Illness* 14:209–16.

Fleming, R. M., 2003 (in press). Angina and coronary ischemia are the results of coronary regional blood flow differences. *J. Amer. Coll. Angiol.*

——. 2001. Coronary artery disease is more than just coronary lumen disease. *Amer. J. Card.* 88:599–600.

——. 2000a. Does routine catheterization and revascularization provide the best results? Preliminary discussion, Annual Amercian College of Cardiology Scientific Sessions, Anaheim, California, March 12.

——. 2000b. Regional blood flow differences induced by high dose dipyridamole explain etiology of angina. Third International College of Coronary Artery Disease from Prevention to Intervention. Lyon, France, October 4.

——. 2000c. Shortcomings of coronary angiography. *Cleve. Clin. J. Med.* 67:450.

Fleming, R. M., L. Boyd, and M. Forster. 2000. Angina is caused by regional blood flow differences; proof of a physiologic (not anatomic) narrowing. Joint session of the European Society of Cardiology and the American College of Cardiology, annual American College of Cardiology Scientific Sessions, Anaheim, California, March 12.

Fleming, R. M., D. M. Fleming, and R. Gaede. 1996. Teaching physicians and health care providers to accurately read coronary arteriograms. *Angiology* 47(4):349–59.

Fleming, R. M., and G. M. Harrington. 1994a. Quantitative coronary arteriography and its assessment of atherosclerosis, part 1: examining the independent variables. *Angiology* 45:829–33.

———. 1994b. Quantitative coronary arteriography and its assessment of atherosclerosis, part 2: calculating stenosis flow reserve directly from percent diameter stenosis. *Angiology* 45:835–40.

Fleming, R. M., R. L. Kirkeeide, R. W. Smalling, et al. 1991. Patterns in visual interpretation of coronary arteriograms as detected by quantitative coronary arteriography. *J. Am. Coll. Cardiol.* 18:945–51.

Foitzik, T., G. Eibl, P. Schneider, et al. 2002. Omega-3 fatty acid supplementation increases anti-inflammatory cytokines and attenuates systemic disease sequelae in experimental pancreatitis. *J. Parenter. Enteral. Nutr.* 26:351–56.

Franke, W. D., S. L. Ramey, and M. C. Shelley. 2002. Relationship between cardiovascular disease morbidity, risk factors, and stress in a law enforcement cohort. *J. Occup. Environ. Med.* 44:1182–89.

Garg, M. L., R. J. Blake, and R. B. Wills. 2003. Macadamia nut consumption lowers plasma total and LDL cholesterol levels in hypercholesterolemic men. *J. Nutr.* 133:1060–63.

Gidron, Y., H. Gilutz, R. Berger, et al. 2002. Molecular and cellular interface between behavior and acute coronary syndromes. *Cardiovasc. Res.* 56:15–21.

Glagov, S., C. K. Zarins, N. Massawa, et al. 1993. Mechanical functional role of non-atherosclerotic intimal thickening. *Front. Med. Biol. Eng.* 5:37–43.

Gould, K. L. 1998a. Coronary arteriography and lipid lowering: limitations, new concepts, and new paradigms in cardiovascular medicine. *Am. J. Cardiol.* 82:12M–21M.

———. 1998b. New concepts and paradigms in cardiovascular medicine: the noninvasive management of coronary artery disease. *Am. J. Med.* 104:2S–17S.

Harvard Heart Letter. June 2002. Coffee and the heart.

Hennekens, C. H. 2002. Update on aspirin in the treatment and prevention of cardiovascular disease. *Am. J. Manag. Care* 8:S691–S700.

Hodge, V. J., S. J. Gould, S. Subramani, et al. 1991. Normal cholesterol synthesis in human cells requires functional peroxisomes. *Biochem. Biophys. Res. Commun.* 181:537–41.

Hu, F. B., E. Cho, K. M. Rexrode, et al. 2003. Fish and long-chain omega-3 fatty acid intake and risk of coronary heart disease and total mortality in diabetic women. *Circulation* 107:1852–57.

Jee, S. H., J. He, L. T. Appel, et al. 2001. Coffee consumption and serum lipids: a meta-analysis of randomized controlled clinical trials. *Am. J. Epidemiol.* 153:353–62.

Keaney, J. F. Jr., M. G. Larson, R. S. Vasan, et al. 2003. Obesity and systemic oxidative stress: clinical correlates of oxidative stress in the Framingham study. *Arterioscler. Thromb. Vasc. Biol.* 23:434–49.

Keys, A., J. T. Anderson, and F. Grande. 1965. Serum cholesterol responses to changes in the diet. The effect of cholesterol in the diet. *Metabolism* 14:759–65.

Koertge, J., F. Al-Khalili, S. Ahnve, et al. 2002. Cortisol and vital exhaustion in relation to significant coronary artery stenosis in middle-aged women with acute coronary syndrome. *Psychoneuroendocrinology* 27:893–906.

Kuper, H., and M. Marmot. 2003. Job strain, job demands, decision latitude, and risk of coronary heart disease within the Whitehall II study. *J. Epidemiol. Community Health* 57:147–53.

Kushi, L., and E. Giovannucci. 2002. Dietary fat and cancer. *Am. J. Med.* 113:63S–70S.

Lovejoy, J. C. 2002. The influence of dietary fat on insulin resistance. *Curr. Diab. Rep.* 2:435–40.

Marinello, E., C. Setacci, M. Giubbolini, et al. 2003. Lipid composition in atheromatous plaque: evolution of the lipid three-phase percentage. *Life Sci.* 72:2689–94.

McMurry, M. P., M. T. Cerqueira, and S. L. Connor, et al. 1991. Changes in lipid and lipoprotein levels and body weight in Tarahumara Indians after consumption of an affluent diet. *New Engl. J. Med.* 325:1704–8.

McMurry, M. P., W. E. Connor, and M. T. Cerqueira. 1982. Dietary cholesterol and the plasma lipids and lipoproteins in the Tarahumara Indians: a people habituated to a low-cholesterol diet after weaning. *Am. J. Clin. Nutr.* 35:741–44.

Ornish, D., L. W. Scherwitz, J. H. Billings, et al. 1998. Intensive lifestyle changes for reversal of coronary heart disease. *JAMA* 280:2001–7.

Petursdottir, D. H., I. Olafsdottir, and I. Hardardottir. 2002. Dietary fish oil increases tumor necrosis factor secretion but decreases interleukin-10 secretion by murine peritoneal macrophages. *J. Nutr.* 132:3740–43.

Radhakrishnan, R., R. Deepa, S. Coimbatore, et al. 2002. Comparison of carotid intima-media thickness, arterial stiffness, and brachial artery flow mediated dilatation in diabetic and nondiabetic subjects (the Chennai Urban Population Study [CUPS-9]). *Am. J. Cardiol.* 90:702–7.

Ridker, P. M., N. Rifai, L. Rose, J. E. Buring, and N. R. Cook. 2002. Comparison of C-reactive protein and low-density lipoprotein cholesterol levels in the prediction of first cardiovascular events. *New Engl. J. Med.* 347(20):1557–65.

Schaffner, T., K. Taylor, E. J. Bartucci, et al. 1980. Arterial foam cells with distinctive immunomorphologic and histochemical features of macrophages. *Am. J. Pathol.* 100:57–80.

Schindler, T. H., B. Hornig, P. T. Buser, et al. 2003. Prognostic value of abnormal vasoreactivity of epicardial coronary arteries to sympathetic stimulation in patients with normal coronary angiograms. *Arterioscler. Thromb. Vasc. Biol.* 23:495–501.

Shoji, T., E. Kimoto, K. Shinohara, et al. 2003. The association of antibodies against oxidized low-density lipoprotein with atherosclerosis in hemodialysis patients. *Kidney Int.* 63:128–30.

Stary, H. C., A. B. Chandler, R. E. Dinsmore, et al. 1995. A definition of advanced types of atherosclerotic lesions and a histological classification of atherosclerosis. A report from the Committee on Vascular Lesions of the

Council on Arteriosclerosis, American Heart Association. *Arterioscler. Thromb. Vasc. Biol.* 15:1512–31.

Stary, H. C., A. B. Chandler, S. Glagov, et al. 1994. A definition of initial, fatty streak, and intermediate lesions of atherosclerosis. A report from the Committee on Vascular Lesions of the Council on Arteriosclerosis, American Heart Association. *Circulation* 89:2462–78.

Stenvinkel, P. 2003. Interactions between inflammation, oxidative stress, and endothelial dysfunction in end-stage renal disease. *J. Ren. Nutr.* 13:144–48.

Steptoe, A., S. Kunz-Ebrecht, A. Rumley, et al. 2003. Prolonged elevations in haemostatic and rheological responses following psychological stress in low socioeconomic status men and women. *Thromb. Haemost.* 89:83–90.

Taylor, K. E., S. Glagov, and C. K. Zarins. 1989. Preservation and structural adaptation of endothelium over experimental foam cell lesions. Quantitative ultrastructural study. *Arteriosclerosis* 9:881–94.

Trichopoulou, A., C. Gnardellis, V. Benetou, et al. 2002. Lipid, protein and carbohydrate intake in relation to body mass index. *Eur. J. Clin. Nutr.* 56:37–43.

Chapter 3: The Truth About Gaining Weight

Butler, R. N., P. August, K. C. Ferdinand, et al. 1999. Hypertension: therapeutic approach to weight loss, exercise and salt intake. *Geriatrics* 54: 45–46, 49–50.

Chu, N. F., J. B. Chang, and S. M. Shieh. 2003. Plasma leptin, fatty acids, and tumor necrosis factor-receptor and insulin resistance in children. *Obes. Res.* 11:532–40.

Dietz, W. H. 1998. Health consequences of obesity in youth: childhood predictors of adult disease. *Pediatrics* 101:518–25.

Engeli, S., P. Schling, K. Gorzelniak, et al. 2003. The adipose-tissue rennin-angiotensin-aldosterone system: role in the metabolic syndrome? *Int. J. Biochem. Cell Biol.* 35:807–25.

Friedman, M., and D. L. Brandon. 2001. Nutritional and health benefits of soy proteins. *J. Agric. Food. Chem.* 49:1069–86.

Ho, J. W., Y. K. Leung, and C. P. Chan. 2002. Herbal medicine in the treatment of cancer. *Curr. Med. Chem. Anti-Canc. Agents* 2:209–14.

Hu, F. B., R. M. van Dam, and S. Liu. 2001. Diet and risk of Type II diabetes: the role of types of fat and carbohydrate. *Diabetologia* 44:805–17.

Jang, J. H., and Y. J. Surh. 2003. Protective effect of resveratrol on beta-amyloid-induced oxidative PC12 cell death. *Free Radic. Biol. Med.* 34:1100–10.

Leonetti, F., G. Lacobellis, A. Zappaterreno, et al. 2002. Clinical, physiopathological and dietetic aspects of metabolic syndrome. *Dig. Liver Dis.* 34:S134–39.

Liu, S., and J. E. Manson. 2001. Dietary carbohydrates, physical inactivity, obesity, and the "metabolic syndrome" as predictors of coronary heart disease. *Curr. Opin. Lipidol.* 12:395–404.

Liu, S., and W. C. Wilett. 2002. Dietary glycemic load and atherothrombotic risk. *Curr. Atheroscler. Rep.* 4:454–61.

Marlett, J. A., M. I. McBurney, and J. L. Slavin. 2002. Position of the American Dietetic Association: health implications of dietary fiber. *J. Am. Diet. Assoc.* 102:993–1000.

Murakami, A., D. Takahashi, K. Koshimizu, et al. 2003. Synergistic suppression of superoxide and nitric oxide generation from inflammatory cells by combined food factors. *Mutat. Res.* 523–24:151–61.

Parihar, M. S., and T. Hemnani. 2003. Phenolic antioxidants attenuate hippocampal neuronal cell damage against kainic acid induced excitotoxicity. *J. Biosci.* 28:121–28.

Pradhan, A. D., N. R. Cook, J. E. Buring, et al. 2003. C-reactive protein is independently associated with fasting insulin in nondiabetic women. *Arterioscler. Thromb. Vasc. Biol.* 23:650–55.

Reaven, G. 2002. Metabolic syndrome: pathophysiology and implications of management of cardiovascular disease. *Circulation* 106:286–88.

Shen, B. J., J. F. Todaro, R. Niaura, et al. 2003. Are metabolic risk factors one unified syndrome? Modeling the structure of the metabolic syndrome X. *Am. J. Epidemiol.* 157:701–11.

Sovak, M. 2001. Grape extract, resveratrol, and its analogs: a review. *J. Med. Food* 4:93–105.

Stoll, Betsy. 1999. Western nutrition and the insulin resistance syndrome: a link to breast cancer. *Eur. J. Clin. Nutr.* 53(2): 83–87.

Truswell, A. S. 2002. Cereal grains and coronary heart disease. *Eur. J. Clin. Nutr.* 56:1–14.

van Dam, R. M., W. C. Willett, E. B. Rimm, et al. 2002. Dietary fat and meat intake in relation to risk of type 2 diabetes in men. *Diabetes Care* 25: 417–24.

Wannamethee, S. Goya, G. A. Shaper, and M. Walker. 2002. Weight change, weight fluctuation, and mortality. *Arch. Intern. Med.* 162(22):2575–80.

Chapter 4: How Exercise Improves Health

Abramson, J. L., and V. Vaccarino. 2002. Relationship between physical activity and inflammation among apparently healthy middle-aged and older U.S. adults. *Arch. Intern. Med.* 162:1286–92.

Abramson, J. L., W. S. Weintraub, and V. Vaccarino. 2002. Association between pulse pressure and C-reactive protein among apparently healthy US adults. *Hypertension.* 39:197.

Banz, W. J., M. A. Maher, W. G. Thompson, et al. 2003. Effects of resistance versus aerobic training on coronary artery disease risk factors. *Exp. Biol. Med.* 228:434–40.

Barbeau, P., M. S. Litaker, K. F. Woods, et al. 2002. Hemostatic and inflammatory markers in obese youths: effects of exercise and adiposity. *J. Pediatr.* 141:415–20.

Barnard, R. J., and S. B. Inkeles. 1999. Effects of an intensive diet and exercise program on lipids in postmenopausal women. *Women's Health Issues* 9:155–61.

Bautista, L. E. 2003. Inflammation, endothelial dysfunction, and the risk of high blood pressure: epidemiologic and biological evidence. *J. Hum. Hypertens.* 17:223–30.

Blair, S. N., H. W. Kohl, R. S. Paffenbarger, D. G. Clark, K. H. Cooper, and L. W. Gibbons. 1989. Physical fitness and all-cause mortality. A prospective study of healthy men and women. *JAMA* 262(17):2395.

Duncan, G. E., M. G. Perri, D. W. Theriaque, et al. 2003. Exercise training, without weight loss, increases insulin sensitivity and postheparin plasma lipase activity in previously sedentary adults. *Diabetes Care* 26:557–62.

Duncan, J. J., N. F. Gordon, and C. B. Scott. 1991. Women walking for health and fitness. How much is enough? *JAMA* 266(23):3295.

Dunn, A. L., B. H. Marcus, J. B. Kampert, et al. 1999. Comparison of lifestyle and structured interventions to increase physical activity and cardiorespiratory fitness. A randomized trial. *JAMA* 281:327–34.

Ford, E. S. 2002. Does exercise reduce inflammation? Physical activity and C-reactive protein among U.S. adults. *Epidemiology* 13:561–68.

Gerardo-Gettens, T., G. D. Miller, B. A. Horwitz, R. B. McDonald, K. D. Bromnel, M. R. Greenwood, J. Rodin, and J. S. Stern. 1991. Exercise decreases fat selection in female rats during weight cycling. *Am. J. Physiol.* 260:R518–24.

Gorman, Christine. "Walk, Don't Run," *Time*, 21 January 2002.

Heald, A., J. Cade, J. Cruickshank, et al. 2003. The influence of dietary intake on the insulin-like growth factor (IGF) system across three ethnic groups: a population-based study. *Public Health Nutr.* 6:175–81.

Horn, P. L., K. Leeman, D. B. Pyne, et al. 2002. Expression of CD94 and 56 (bright) on natural killer lymphocytes—the influence of exercise. *International J. Sports. Med.* 23:595–99.

Isasi, C. R., R. J. Deckelbaum, R. P. Tracy, et al. 2003. Physical fitness and C-reactive protein level in children and young adults: the Columbia University BioMarkers Study. *Pediatrics* 111:332–38.

King, D. E., P. Carek, A. G. Mainous, et al. 2003. Inflammatory markers and exercise: differences related to exercise type. *Med. Sci. Sports Exerc.* 35:575–81.

Koutsari, C., F. Karpe, S. M. Humphreys, et al. 2001. Exercise prevents the accumulation of triglyceride-rich lipoproteins and their remnants seen when changing to a high-carbohydrate diet. *Arterioscler. Thromb. Vasc. Biol.* 21:1520–25.

Kraus, W. E., J. A. Houmard, B. D. Duscha, et al. 2002. Effects of the amount and intensity of exercise on plasma lipoproteins. *New Engl. J. Med.* 347:1483–92.

LaMonte, Michael J. 2002. Cardiorespiratory fitness and C-reactive protein among a tri-ethnic sample of women. *Circulation* 106(4):403–6.

Ma, J., Z. Liu, and W. Ling. 2003. Physical activity, diet and cardiovascular disease risks in Chinese women. *Public Health Nutr.* 6:139–47.

Manchanda, S. C., R. Narang, K. S. Reddy, et al. 2000. Retardation of coronary atherosclerosis with yoga lifestyle intervention. *J. Assoc. Physicians India* 48:687–94.

McLaughlin, T., F. Abbasi, C. Lamendola, et al. 2002. Differentiation between obesity and insulin resistance in the association with C-reactive protein. *Circulation* 106:2908–12.

Metzler, B., R. Abia, M. Ahmad, et al. 2003. Activation of heat shock transcription factor 1 in atherosclerosis. *Am. J. Pathol.* 162:1669–76.

Paffenbarger, R. S., R. T. Hyde, A. L. Wing, I-Min Lee, D. L. Jung, and J. B. Kampert. 1993. The association of change in physical activity level and other lifestyle characteristics with mortality among men. *New Engl. J. Med.* 328:538–45.

Pedersen, B. K., A. Steensberg, P. Keller, et al. 2003. Muscle-derived interleukin-6: lipolytic, anti-inflammatory and immune regulatory effects. *Pflugers Arch.* 446:9–16.

Sandvik, L., J. Erikssen, E. Thaulow, E. Gunnar, R. Mundal, and K. Rodahl. 1993. Physical fitness as a predictor of mortality among healthy, middle-aged Norwegian men. *New Engl. J. Med.* 328:533–37.

Shepard, R. 2003. Adhesion molecules, catecholamines and leucocyte redistribution during and following exercise. *Sports Med.* 33:261–84.

Simoes, E. J., T. Byers, R. J. Coates, M. K. Serdula, A. H. Mokdad, and G. W. Heath. 1995. The association between leisure-time physical activity and dietary fat in American adults. *Am. J. of Pub. Health* 85(2): 240–44.

Tanasescu, M., M. F. Leitzmann, E. B. Rimm, et al. 2002. Exercise type and intensity in relation to coronary heart disease in men. *JAMA* 288: 1994–2000.

Taylor-Piliae, R. E. 2003. Tai chi as an adjunct to cardiac rehabilitation exercise training. *J. Cardiopulm. Rehabil.* 23:90–96.

Thune, I. 1997. Physical activity and the risk of breast cancer. *New Engl. J. Med.* 336:1269.

Wannamethee, S. G., G. Lowe, P. H. Whincup, A. Rumley, M. Walker, and L. Lennon. 2002. Physical activity and hemostatic and inflammatory variables in elderly men. *Circulation* 105:1785.

Wood, P. D., R. B. Terry, and W. I. Haskell. 1985. Metabolism of substrates: diet, lipoprotein metabolism, and exercise. *Fed. Proc.* 44:358–63.

Yan, H., A. Kuroiwa, H. Tanaka, et al. 2001. Effect of moderate exercise on immune senescence in men. *Eur. J. Appl. Physiol.* 86:105–11.

Zheng, W., X. O. Shu, J. K. McLaughlin, et al. 1993. Occupational physical activity and the risk of cancers of the breast, corpus uteri and ovary. *Cancer* 71:3670–4.

Chapter 5: Homocysteine and Antioxidants

Abu-Khader, A. A., and Y. Y. Bilto. 2002. Exposure of human neutrophils to oxygen radicals causes loss of deformity, lipid peroxidation, protein degradation, respiratory burst activation and loss of migration. *Clin. Hemorheol. Microcirc.* 27:57–66.

Alho, H., J. S. Leinonen, M. Erhola, et al. 1998. Assay of antioxidant capacity of human plasma and CSF in aging and disease. *Restor. Neurol. Neurosci.* 12:159–65.

Annuk, M., M. Zilmer, and B. Fellstrom. 2003. Endothelium-dependent vasodilation and oxidative stress in chronic renal failure: impact on cardiovascular disease. *Kidney Int. Suppl.* 84:50–53.

Bickford, P. C., T. Gould, L. Briederick, et al. 2000. Antioxidant-rich diets improve cerebellar physiology and motor learning in aged rats. *Brain Res.* 866:211–17.

Bollinger, W. S., T. J. Babineau, and G. L. Blackburn. 1998. Nutrition notes. The antioxidant vitamins. *Contem. Intern. Med.* 10:44–47.

Chambers, J. C., A. McGregor, J. Jean-Marie, et al. 1998. Acute hyperhomocysteinaemia and endothelial dysfunction. *Lancet* 351:36–37.

Das, U. N. 1998. Oxidants, antioxidants, essential fatty acids, eicosanoids, cytokines, gene/oncogene expression and apoptosis in systemic lupus erythematosus. *J. Assoc. Physicians India* 46:630–34.

El-Khairy, L., S. E. Vollset, H. Refsum, et al. 2003. Plasma total cysteine, pregnancy complications, and adverse pregnancy outcomes: the Hordaland Homocysteine Study. *Am. J. Clin. Nutr.* 77:467–72.

Fitzpatrick, D. F., B. Bing, D. A. Maggi, et al. 2002. Vasodilating procyanidins derived from grape seeds. *Ann. N.Y. Acad. Sci.* 957:78–89.

Fleming, R. M. 2003. The influence of diet on homocysteine. Fourth International Homocysteine Conference, Basel, Switzerland, June.

Fonseca, V., A. Dicker-Brown, S. Ranganathan, et al. 2000. Effects of a high-fat-sucrose diet on enzymes in homocysteine metabolism in the rat. *Metabolism* 49:736–41.

Jiang, X. C., A. R. Tall, S. Qin, et al. 2002. Phospholipid transfer protein deficiency protects circulating lipoproteins from oxidation due to the enhanced accumulation of vitamin E. *J. Biol. Chem.* 277:31850–56.

Kluijtmans, L. A., I. S. Young, C. A. Boreham, et al. 2003. Genetic and nutritional factors contributing to hyperhomocysteinemia in young adults. *Blood* 101:2483–88.

Knight, D. C., and J. A. Eden. 1996. A review of the clinical effects of phytoestrogens. *Obstet. Gynecol.* 87:897–904.

Laugesen, M., and R. Elliott. 2003. Ischaemic heart disease, Type 1 diabetes, and cow milk A1 beta-casein. *N. Z. Med. J.* 116:U295.

McCully, K. S. 1998. The homocysteine revolution: medicine in the new millennium; beyond cholesterol: the homocysteine theory of arteriosclerosis. Parts 1 & 2. *Cardiovasc. Rev. & Rep.* 30–45; 57–65.

Mikhov, D., P. Markova, and R. Girchev. 1998. Spectral analysis of heart rate and arterial pressure variability after nitric oxide synthase inhibition. *Acta Physiol. Pharmacol. Bulg.* 23:79–84.

Morita, H., H. Kurihara, S. Yoshida, et al. 2001. Diet-induced hyperhomocysteinemia exacerbates neointima formation in rat carotid arteries after balloon injury. *Circulation* 103:133–39.

Okatani, Y., A. Wakatsuki, and R. J. Reiter. 2000. Protective effect of melatonin against homocysteine-induced vasoconstriction of human unbilical artery. *Biochem. Bioph. Res. Co.* 277:470–75.

Orzechowski, A. 2003. Justification for antioxidant preconditioning (or how to protect insulin-mediated actions under oxidative stress). *J. Biosci.* 28: 39–49.

Pathak, S. K., R. A. Sharma, and J. K. Mellon. 2003. Chemoprevention of prostate cancer by diet-derived antioxidant agents and hormonal manipulation (review). *Int. J. Oncol.* 22:5–13.

Retterstol, L., B. Paus, M. Bohn, et al. 2003. Plasma homocysteine levels and prognosis in patients with previous premature myocardial infarction: a 10-year follow-up study. *J. Intern. Med.* 253:284–92.

Rowling, M. J., M. H. McMullen, D. C. Chipman, et al. 2002. Hepatic glycine N-methyltransferase is up-regulated by excess dietary methionine in rats. *J. Nutr.* 132:2545–50.

Seshadri, S., A. Beiser, J. Selhub, et al. 2002. Plasma homocysteine as a risk factor for dementia and Alzheimer's disease. *New Engl. J. Med.* 346:476–83.

Solfrizzi, V., F. Panza, and A. Capurso. 2003. The role of diet in cognitive decline. *J. Neural. Transm.* 110:95–110.

Spieker, L. E., I. Sudano, D. Hurlimann, et al. 2002. High-density lipoprotein restores endothelial function in hypercholesterolemic men. *Circulation* 105:1399–402.

Tham, D. M., C. D. Gardner, and W. L. Haskell. 1998. Clinical review 97. Potential health benefits of dietary phytoestrogens: a review of the clinical, epidemiological, and mechanistic evidence. *J. Clin. Endocrinol. Metab.* 83:2223–35.

Tyagi, S C. 1999. Homocyst(e)ine and heart disease: pathophysiology of extracellular matrix. *Clin. Exp. Hypertens.* 21:181–98.

Tyagi, S. C., L. M. Smiley, V. S. Mujumdar, et al. 1998. Reduction oxidation (Redox) and vascular tissue level of homocyst(e)ine in human coronary artherosclerotic lesions and role in extracellular matrix remodeling and vascular tone. *Mol. Cell. Biochem.* 181:107–16.

Ureland, P. M., O. Nygard, S. E. Vollset, et al. 2001. The Hordaland Homocysteine studies. *Lipids* 36:S33–39.

Ungvari, Z., and A. Koller. 2001. Homocysteine reduces smooth muscle [Ca2+]I and constrictor responses of isolated arterioles. *J. Cardiovasc. Pharmacol.* 37:705–12.

Weiss, N., Y. Y. Zhang, S. Heydrick, et al. 2001. Overexpression of cellular glutathione peroxidase rescues homocyst(e)ine-induced endothelial dysfunction. *Proc. Natl. Acad. Sci. USA* 98:12503–8.

Willett, Walter, et al. 2001. Types of dietary fat and risk of coronary heart disease: a critical review. *J. Am. Coll. Nutr.* 20(1):5–19.

Chapter 6: Growth Factors, Fibrinogen, and Lipoprotein (a)

Abramson, J. L., V. Vaccarino. 2002. Relationship between physical activity and inflammation among apparently healthy middle-aged and older U.S. adults. *Arch. Intern. Med.* 162(11):1286–92.

Aguejouf, O., K. Mayo, L. Monteiro, et al. 2002. Increase of arterial thrombosis parameters in chronic *Helicobacter pylori* infection in mice. *Thromb. Res.* 108:245–48.

Armstrong, V. W., A. K. Walli, and D. Seidel. 1985. Isolation, characterization, and uptake in human fibroblasts of an apo(a)-free lipoprotein obtained on reduction of lipoprotein (a). *J. Lipid Res.* 26:1314–23.

Banz, W. J., M. A. Maher, W. G. Thompson, et al. 2003. Effects of resistance versus aerobic training on coronary artery disease risk factors. *Exp. Biol. Med.* 228:434–40.

Birgisdottir, B. E., J. P. Hill, D. P. Harris, et al. 2002. Variation in consumption of cow milk proteins and lower incidence of Type 1 diabetes in Iceland vs the other four Nordic countries. *Diabetes Nutr. Metab.* 15:240–45.

Champion, Z. J., E. A. James, M. H. Vickers, et al. 2000. The effects of bovine recombinant growth hormone administration on insulin-like growth factor-1 and the haemopoietic system in Thoroughbred geldings. *Vet. J.* 160:147–52.

Chang, S., X. Wu, H. Yu, et al. 2002. Plasma concentrations of insulin-like growth factors among healthy adult men and postmenopausal women: associations with body composition, lifestyle, and reproductive factors. *Cancer Epidemiol. Biomarkers Prev.* 11:758–66.

Decensi, A., U. Omodei, C. Robertson, et al. 2002. Effect of transdermal estradiol and oral conjugated estrogen on C-reactive protein in retinoid-placebo trial in healthy women. *Circulation* 106:1224–28.

Emanuele, N., N. Azad, C. Abraira, et al. 1998. Effect of intensive glycemic control on fibrinogen, lipids, and lipoproteins. Veterans Affairs Cooperative Study in type II diabetes mellitus. *Arch. Intern. Med.* 158:2485–90.

Epstein, S. S. 1996. Unlabeled milk from cows treated with biosynthetic growth hormones: a case of regulatory abdication. *International J. Health Serv.* 26:173–85.

Folmar, S., F. Oates-Williams, P. Sharp, et al. 2001. Recruitment of participants for the Estrogen Replacement and Atherosclerosis (ERA) trial, a comparison of costs, yields, and participant characteristics from community- and hospital-based recruitment strategies. *Control Clin. Trials* 22: 13–25.

Gaw, A., G. Docherty, and E. A. Brown. 1999. Predictors of plasma lipoprotein (a) concentration in the West of Scotland Coronary Prevention Study cohort. *Atherosclerosis* 143:445–50.

Grady, D., D. Herrington, V. Bittner, et al. 2002. Cardiovascular disease outcomes during 6.8 years of hormonal therapy: Heart and Estrogen/progestin Replacement Study follow-up (HERS II). *JAMA* 288:99–101.

Haffner, S. M., K. K. Gruber, P. A. Morales, et al. 1992. Lipoprotein (a) concentrations in Mexican Americans and non-Hispanic whites: the San Antonio Heart Study. *Am. J. Epidemiol.* 136:1060–68.

Hall, J. L., G. H. Gibbons, and J. C. Chatham. 2002. IGF-1 promotes a shift in metabolic flux in vascular smooth muscle cells. *Am. J. Physiol. Endocrinol. Metab.* 283:E465–71.

Holme, I., P. Urdal, S. Anderssen, et al. 1996. Exercise-induced increase in lipoprotein (a). *Atherosclerosis* 122:97–104.

Hulley, S. 2000. Estrogens should not be initiated for the secondary prevention of coronary artery disease: a debate. *Can. J. Cardiol,* Suppl. E:10E–12E.

Hulley, S., C. Furberg, E. Barrett-Connor, et al. 2002. Noncardiovascular disease outcomes during 6.8 years of hormone therapy: Heart and Estrogen/progestin Replacement Study follow-up (HERS II). *JAMA* 288: 58–66.

Hulley, S., D. Grady, T. Bush, et al. 1998. Randomized trial of estrogen plus progestin for secondary prevention of coronary heart disease in post-menopausal women. Heart and Estrogen/progestin Replacement Study (HERS) Research Group. *JAMA* 280:605–13.

Inoue, K., N. Nago, H. Matsuo, et al. 1997. Serum insulin and lipoprotein (a) concentrations. The Jichi Medical School Cohort Study. *Diabetes Care* 20:1242–47.

Jaber, J., J. Murin, S. Kinova, et al. 2002. The role of infection and inflammation in the pathogenesis of atherosclerosis. *Vnitr. Lek.* 48:657–66.

Jenner, J. L., J. M. Ordovas, S. Lamon-Fava, et al. 1993. Effects of age, sex, and menopausal status on plasma lipoprotein (a) levels. The Framingham Offspring Study. *Circulation* 87:1135–41.

Juul, A., T. Scheike, M. Davidsen, et al. 2002. Low serum insulin-like growth factor I is associated with increased risk of ischemic heart disease: a population-based case-control study. *Circulation* 106:939–44.

Karjalainen, J., J. M. Martin, M. Knip, J. Ilonen, B. H. Robinson, E. Savilahti, H. K. Akerblom, and H. M. Dosch. 1992. A bovine albumin peptide as a possible trigger of insulin-dependent diabetes mellitus. *New Engl. J. Med.* 327:302–7.

Kaysen, G. A., and V. Kumar. 2003. Inflammation in ESRD: causes and potential consequences. *J. Ren. Nutr.* 13:158–60.

King, D. E., P. Carek, A. D. Mainous, et al. 2003. Inflammatory markers and exercise: differences related to exercise type. *Med. Sci. Sports Exerc.* 35:575–81.

Kluft, C., J. A. Leuven, F. M. Helmerhorst, et al. 2002. Pro-inflammatory effects of oestrogens during use of oral contraceptives and hormone replacement treatment. *Vascul. Pharmacol.* 39:149–54.

Lako, J. V., and V. C. Nguyen. 2001. Dietary patterns and risk factors of diabetes mellitus among urban indigenous women in Fiji. *Asia Pac. J. Clin. Nutr.* 10:188–93.

Laugesen, M., and R. Elliott. 2003. Ischaemic heart disease, Type 1 diabetes, and cow milk A1 beta-casein. *N. Z. Med. J.* 116:U295.

Levitsky, L. L., A. M. Scanu, and S. H. Gould. 1991. Lipoprotein (a) levels in black and white children and adolescents with IDDM. *Diabetes Care* 14:283–87.

Longo, V. D., and P. Fabrizio. 2002. Regulation of longevity and stress resistance: a molecular strategy conserved from yeast to humans? *Cell. Mol. Life Sci.* 59:903–8.

Lunt, M., P. Masaryk, C. Scheidt-Nave, et al. 2001. The effects of lifestyle, dietary dairy intake and diabetes on bone density and vertebral deformity prevalence: the EVOS study. *Osteoporos.* 12:688–98.

Mandelbaum-Schmid, J. 1998. Detecting heart disease. *Hippocrates.*

Martin, S., R. R. Elosua, M. I. Covas, M. Pavesi, J. Vila, and J. Marrugat. 1999. Relationship of lipoprotein(a) levels to physical activity and family history of coronary heart disease. *Am. J. Public Health* 89:856–61.

McLachlan, C. N. 2001. Beta-casein A1, ischaemic heart disease mortality, and other illnesses. *Med. Hypotheses* 56:262–72.

Nago, N., K. Kayaba, and J. Hiraoka, et al. 1995. Lipoprotein (a) levels in the Japanese population: influence of age and sex, and relation to atherosclerotic risk factors. The Jichi Medical School Cohort Study. *Am. J. Epidemiol.* 141:815–21.

Pradhan, A. D., J. E. Manson, J. E. Rossouw, et al. 2002. Inflammatory biomarkers, hormone replacement therapy, and incident coronary heart disease: prospective analysis from the Women's Health Initiative observational study. *JAMA* 288:980–87.

Rakic, V., I. B. Puddey, S. B. Dimmitt, et al. 1998. A controlled trial of the effects of pattern of alcohol intake on serum lipid levels in regular drinkers. *Atherosclerosis* 137:243–52.

Ramirez-Bosca, A., A. Soler, M. A. Carrion-Gutierrez, et al. 2000. An hydroalcoholic extract of *Curcuma longa* lowers the abnormally high values of human-plasma fibrinogen. *Mech. Ageing Dev.* 114(3):207–10.

Randal, J. 2002. The end of an era? Study reveals harms of hormone replacement therapy. *J. Natl. Cancer Inst.* 94:1116–18.

Retzinger, G. S. 2002. Fibrinogen-coated chylomicrons in gastrointestinal lymph: a new rationale regarding the arterial deposition of postprandial lipids. *Med. Hypotheses* 59:718–26.

Schachinger, V., M. Haller, J. Minners, et al. 1997. Lipoprotein (a) selectively impairs receptor-mediated endothelial vasodilator function of the human coronary circulation. *J. Am. Coll. Cardiol.* 30:927–34.

Selby, J. V., M. A. Austin, C. Sandholzer, et al. 1994. Environmental and behavioral influences on plasma lipoprotein (a) concentration in women twins. *Prev. Med.* 23:345–53.

Selvais, P., J. Henrion, M. Schapira, et al. 1995. Lipoprotein (a) in liver diseases. Correlation between low levels and liver function. *Presse Med.* 24:382–86.

Shah, S. H., and K. P. Alexander. 2003. Hormone replacement therapy for primary and secondary prevention of heart disease. *Curr. Treat. Options Cardiovasc. Med.* 5:25–33.

Shen, W. H., J. H. Zhou, S. R. Broussard, et al. 2002. Pro-inflammatory cytokines block growth of breast cancer cells by impairing signals from a growth factor receptor. *Cancer Res.* 62:4746–56.

Simmons, J. G., J. B. Pucilowska, T. O. Keku, et al. 2002. IGF-1 and TGF-beta have distinct effects on phenotype and proliferation of intestinal fibroblasts. *Am. J. Physiol. Gastrointest. Liver Physiol.* 283:G809–18.

Stein, J. H., and P. E. McBride. 1999. Screening and managing patients with lipoprotein (a) excess. *Internal Med.* 20:9–21.

Takahashi, S., T. Yamamoto, Y. Moriwaki, et al. 1995. Increased concentrations of serum Lp(a) lipoprotein in patients with primary gout. *Ann. Rheum. Dis.* 54:90–93.

Wassef, G. N. 1999. Lipoprotein (a) in android obesity and NIDDM: a new member in the "metabolic syndrome." *Biomed. Pharmacother.* 53:462–65.

Weng, X., G. O. Roederer, R. Beaulieu, et al. 1998. Contribution of acute-phase proteins and cardiovascular risk factors to erythrocytes aggregation in normolipidemic and hyperlipidemic individuals. *Thromb. Haemost.* 80:903–8.

Women's Health Initiative Study Group. 1998. Design of the Women's Health Initiative clinical trial and observational study. *Control Clin. Trials* 19:61–109.

Writing Group for the Women's Health Initiative Investigators. 2002. Risks and benefits of estrogen plus progestin in healthy postmenopausal women. Principal results from the Women's Health Initiative Randomized Controlled Trial. *JAMA* 288:321–33.

Ylikorkala, O., and M. Metsa-Heikkila. 2002. Hormone replacement therapy in women with a history of breast cancer. *Gynecol. Endocrinol.* 16:469–78.

Zanger, D., B. K. Yang, J. Ardans, et al. 2000. Divergent effects of hormone therapy on serum markers of inflammation in postmenopausal women with coronary artery disease on appropriate medical management. *J. Am. Coll. Cardiol.* 36:1797–802.

Zhang, X., and D. Yee. 2002. Insulin-like growth factor binding protein-1 (IGFBP-1) inhibits breast cancer cell motility. *Cancer Res.* 62:4369–75.

Chapter 7: Leukotrienes, Complement, and Bacteria

Aggarwall, B. B., A. Kumar, and A. C. Bharti. 2003. Anticancer potential of curcumin: preclinical and clinical studies. *Nat. Lib. of Med.* 23(1A): 363–98.

Akoachere, J. F., R. N. Ndip, E. B. Chenwi, et al. 2002. Antibacterial effect of *Zingiber officinale* and *Garcinia kola* on respiratory tract pathogens. *East Afr. Med. J.* 79:588–92.

Allen, S., M. Dashwood, K. Morrison, et al. 1998. Differential leukotrienes constrictor responses in human atherosclerotic coronary arteries. *Circulation* 97:2406–13.

Barrett, T. D., J. K. Hennan, R. M. Marks, et al. 2002. C-reactive-protein—associated increase in myocardial infarct size after ischemia/reperfusion. *J. Pharmacol. Exp. Ther.* 303:1007–13.

Bottiger, B. W., J. Motsch, V. Braun, et al. 2002. Marked activation of complement and leukocytes and an increase in the concentrations of soluble endothelial adhesion molecules during cardiopulmonary resuscitation and early reperfusion after cardiac arrest in humans. *Crit. Care Med.* 30:2473–80.

Brunner, E. J., H. Hemingway, B. R. Walker, et al. 2002. Adrenocortical, autonomic, and inflammatory causes of the metabolic syndrome: nested case-control study. *Circulation* 106:2659–65.

Bullo, M., P. Garcia-Lorda, I. Megias, et al. 2003. Systemic inflammation, adipose tissue tumor necrosis factor, and leptin expression. *Obes. Res.* 11:525–31.

Chainani-Wu, N. 2003. Safety and anti-inflammatory activity of curcumin: a component of tumeric (*Curcuma longa*). *J. Altern. Complement. Med.* 9:161–68.

Elenkov, I. J., and G. P. Chrousos. 2002. Stress hormones, pro-inflammatory and anti-inflammatory cytokines, and autoimmunity. *Ann. N.Y. Acad. Sci.* 966:290–303.

Eriksson, U., M. O. Kurrer, N. Schmitz, et al. 2003. Interleukin-6–deficient mice resist development of autoimmune myocarditis associated with impaired up-regulation of complement C3. *Circulation* 107:320–25.

Esposito, K., A. Pontillo, C. Di Palo, et al. 2003. Effect of weight loss and lifestyle changes on vascular inflammatory markers in obese women: a randomized trial. *JAMA* 289:1799–804.

Fleming, R. M. 2003 (in press). Using C-reactive protein as a marker of bacterially aggravated atherosclerosis in acute coronary syndromes. *J. Amer. Coll. Angiol.*

——. 2000. The Fleming Unified Theory of vascular disease. A link between atherosclerosis, inflammation, and bacterially aggravated atherosclerosis (BAA). *Angiology* 51:87–89.

Gebert, A., D. Behrend, G. Zinner, et al. 2002. Comparative analysis of in vitro test procedures for evaluating hemocompatibility of cardiovascular stents. *Biomed. Tech.* 47:827–30.

Gould, J. M., and J. N. Weiser. 2001. Expression of C-reactive protein in the human respiratory tract. *Infect. Immun.* 69:1747–54.

Grabie, N., M. W. Delfs, J. R. Westrich, et al. 2003. IL-12 is required for differentiation of pathogenic CD8+ T cell effectors that cause myocarditis. *J. Clin. Invest.* 111:671–80.

Hack, C. E. 2002. CRP and cardiovascular disease: Linked by complement? *Neth. J. Med.* 60:297–98.

Halvorsen, B. L., K. Holte, M. C. Myhrstad, et al. 2002. A systemic screening of total antioxidants in dietary plants. *J. Nutr.* 132:461–71.

Heinz, A., D. Hermann, M. N. Smolka, et al. 2003. Effects of acute psychological stress on adhesion molecules, interleukins and sex hormones: implications for coronary heart disease. *Psychopharmacology* 165:111–17.

Hiki, N., Y. Mimura, F. Hatao, et al. 2003. Sublethal endotoxin administration evokes super-resistance to systemic hypoxia in rats. *J. Trauma* 54: 584–89.

Horstick, G. 2002. C1-esterase inhibitor in ischemia and reperfusion. *Immunobiology* 205:552–62.

Jensen, E., S. Andreasson, A. Bengtsson, et al. 2003. Influence of two different perfusion systems on inflammatory responses in pediatric heart surgery. *Ann. Thorac. Surg.* 75:919–25.

Legssyer, A., A. Ziyyat, H. Mekhfi, et al. 2002. Cardiovascular effects of *Urtica dioica L.* in isolated rat heart and aorta. *Phytother. Res.* 16:503–7.

Lim, A. G., C. Walker, S. Chambers, et al. 1997. *Helicobacter pylori* eradication using a seven-day regimen of low-dose clarithromycin, lansoprazole and amoxycillin. *Aliment Pharmacol. Ther.* 11:1001–2.

Lvey, J. H., and K. A. Tanaka. 2003. Inflammatory response to cardiopulmonary bypass. *Ann. Thorac. Surg.* 75:S715–20.

Martin, S., R. Elosua, M. I. Covas, M. Pavesi, J. Vila, and J. Marrugat. 1999. Relationship of lipoprotein (a) levels to physical activity and family history of coronary heart disease. *Amer. Jour. of Pub. Health* 89(3):383.

May, A. E., V. Redecke, S. Grüner, et al. 2003. Recruitment of *Chlamydia pneumoniae*–infected macrophages to the carotid artery wall in non-infected nonatherosclerotic mice. *Arter., Throm., and Vasc. Biol.* 23:789.

Mendall, M. A., P. M. Goggia, N. Molineaux, et al. 1994. Relation of *Helicobacter pylori* infection and coronary heart disease. *Br. Heart. J.* 71: 437–39.

Miller, G. E., C. A. Stetler, R. M. Carney, et al. 2002. Clinical depression and inflammatory risk markers for coronary heart disease. *Am. J. Cardiol.* 90:1279–83.

Oral, H., N. Sivasubramanian, B. D. Dyke, et al. 2003. Myocardial pro-inflammatory cytokine expression and left ventricular remodeling in patients with chronic mitral regurgitation. *Circulation* 107:831–37.

Parissis, J. T., S. Adamopoulos, K. F. Venetsanou, et al. 2002. Serum profiles of C-C chemokines in acute myocardial infarction: possible implications in post-infarction left ventricular remodeling. *J. Interferon Cytokine Res.* 22:223–29.

Reuters Health Information. 2003. U.S. smallpox vaccine campaign linked with 45 serious adverse events. *Morbidity and Mortality Weekly Report* 52:360–63. Also at www.medscape.com.

Rodbard, S., and C. Yamamoto. 1969. Effect of stream velocity on bacterial deposition and growth. *Cardiovasc. Res.* 3:68–74.

Rossi, P., P. Kuukasjarvi, J. P. Salenius, et al. 1997. Leukotriene production is increased in lower limb ischemia. *Intern. J. Angiol.* 6:89–90.

Roubenoff, R. 2003. Catabolism of aging: Is it an inflammatory process? *Curr. Opin. Clin. Nutr. Metab. Care* 6:295–99.

Shamsuzzaman, A. S., M. Winnicki, P. Lanfranchi, et al. 2002. Elevated C-reactive protein in patients with obstructive sleep apnea. *Circulation* 105:2462–64.

Spencer, L. 2002. Results of a heart disease risk-factor screening among traditional college students. *J. Am. Coll. Health* 50:291–96.

Stinson, M. W., S. Alder, and S. Kumar. 2003. Invasion and killing of human endothelial cells by viridans group streptococci. *Infect. Immun.* 71:2365–72.

Suzuki, M., S. Inaba, T. Nagai, et al. 2003. Relation of C-reactive protein and interleukin-6 to culprit coronary artery plaque size in patients with acute myocardial infarction. *Am. J. Cardiol.* 91:331–33.

Testai, L., S. Chericoni, V. Calderone, et al. 2002. Cardiovascular effects of *Urtica dioica L.* (*Urticaceae*) roots extracts: in vitro and in vivo pharmacological studies. *J. Ethnopharmacol.* 81:105–9.

Vasan, R. S., L. M. Sullivan, R. Roubenoff, et al. 2003. Inflammatory markers and risk of heart failure in elderly subjects without prior myocardial infarction: the Framingham Heart Study. *Circulation* 107:1486–91.

Wharton, M., R. A. Strikas, R. Harpaz, et al. 2003. Recommendations for using smallpox vaccine in a pre-event vaccination program. Supplemental recommendations of the Advisory Committee on Immunization Practices (ACIP) and the Healthcare Infection Control Practices Advisory Committee (HICPAC). *Morbidity and Mortality Weekly Report Recomm. Rep.* 52:1–16.

Yamashita, H., K. Shimada, E. Seki, et al. 2003. Concentrations of interleukins, interferon, and C-reactive protein in stable and unstable angina pectoris. *Am. J. Cardiol.* 91:133–36.

Yokoe, T., K. Minoguchi, H. Matsuo, et al. 2003. Elevated levels of C-reactive protein and interleukin-6 in patients with obstructive sleep apnea syndrome are decreased by nasal continuous positive airway pressure. *Circulation* 107:1129–34.

Ziccardi, P., F. Nappo, G. Giugliano, et al. 2002. Reduction of inflammatory cytokine concentrations and improvement of endothelial functions in obese women after weight loss over one year. *Circulation* 105:804–9.

Zoccali, C., F. Mallamaci, and G. Tripepi. 2003. Adipose tissue as a source of inflammatory cytokines in health and disease: focus on end-stage renal disease. *Kidney Int. Suppl.* 84:65–68.

Zwaka, T. P., D. Manolov, C. Ozdemir, et al. 2002. Complement and dilated cardiomyopathy: a role of sublytic terminal complement complex-induced tumor necrosis factor-alpha synthesis in cardiac myocytes. *Am. J. Pathol.* 161:449–57.

Chapter 8: Protect Your Arteries

Beauman, G. J., and R. A. Vogel. 1990. Accuracy of individual and panel interpretations of coronary arteriograms: implications for clinical decisions. *J. Am. Coll. Cardiol.* 16:108–13.

Belhassen, L., G. Pelle, J. L. Dubois-Rande, et al. 2003. Improved endothelial function by the thromboxane A2 receptor antagonist S 18886 in patients with coronary artery disease treated with aspirin. *J. Am. Coll. Cardiol.* 41:1198–1204.

Biasucci, L. M., M. Santamaria, and G. Liuzzo. 2002. Inflammation, atherosclerosis and acute coronary syndromes. *Minerva Cardioangiol.* 50: 475–86.

Bonow, R. O., and S. E. Epstein. 1985. Indications for coronary artery bypass surgery in patients with chronic angina pectoris: implications of the multicenter randomized trials. *Circulation* 72:V23–30.

Burke, A. P., A. Farb, G. T. Malcom, et al. 1999. Plaque rupture and sudden death related to exertion in men with coronary artery disease. *JAMA* 281:921–26.

Caracciolo, E. A., K. B. Davis, G. Sopko, et al. 1995. Comparison of surgical and medical group survival in patients with left main equivalent coronary artery disease. Long-term CASS experience. *Circulation* 91:2335–44.

Chan, A. W., D. L. Bhatt, D. P. Chew, et al. 2003. Relation of inflammation and benefit of statins after percutaneous coronary interventions. *Circulation* 107:1750–56.

Chenevard, R., D. Hurlimann, M. Bechir, et al. 2003. Selective COX-2 inhibition improves endothelial function in coronary artery disease. *Circulation* 107:405–9.

Dake, M. 2001. Recombinant VEGF may have atherosclerotic side effects. *Nature Med.* 7:403–4.

Davis, K. B., L. Fisher, and M. Pettinger. 1985. The effect of clinical characteristics on the comparison of medical and surgical therapy in the Coronary Artery Surgery Study (CASS) and the Veterans Administration Cooperative trial. *Circulation* 72:V117–22.

DeBruyne, B., F. Hersbach, N. H. Pijls, et al. 2001. Abnormal epicardial coronary resistance in patients with diffuse atherosclerosis but "normal" coronary angiography. *Circulation* 104:2401–6.

DeRouen, T. A., J. A. Murphy, and W. Owen. 1977. Variability in the analysis of coronary arteriograms. *Circulation* 55:324–28.

Detre, K. M., E. Wright, M. L. Murphy, et al. 1975. Agreement in evaluation coronary angiograms. *Circulation* 52:979–86.

Espinola-Klein, C., H. J. Rupprecht, R. Erbel, et al. 2000. Ten-year outcome after coronary angioplasty in patients with single-vessel coronary artery disease and comparison with the results of the Coronary Artery Surgery Study (CASS). *Am. J. Cardiol.* 85:321–26.

Fischell, T. A., G. Derby, T. M. Tse, et al. 1988. Coronary artery vasoconstriction routinely occurs after percutaneous transluminal coronary angioplasty: a quantitative arteriographic analysis. *Circ. J. Am. Heart Assoc.* 78:1323–34.

Fleming, R. M. 2002a. High-dose dipyridamole and gated sestamibi SPECT imaging provide diagnostic resting and stress ejection fractions useful for predicting the extent of coronary artery disease. *Angiology* 53:415–21.

———. 2002b. A tate-en-tate comparison of ejection fraction and regional wall motion abnormalities as measured by echocardiography and gated sestamibi SPECT. *Angiology* 53:313–21.

———. 2001. Coronary artery disease is more than just coronary lumen disease. *Am. J. Cardiol.* 88:599–600.

———. 2000. Regional blood flow differences induced by high dose dipyridamole explain etiology of angina. Third International College of Coronary Artery Disease from Prevention to Intervention. Lyon, France, October 4.

———. 1999. Atherosclerosis. Understanding the relationship between coronary artery disease and stenosis flow reserve. In *Textbook of Angiology*, ed. John C. Chang, pp. 381–87. New York: Springer-Verlag.

Fleming, R. M., L. Boyd, and M. Forster. 2000. Angina is caused by regional blood flow differences—proof of a physiologic (not anatomic) narrowing. Joint Session of the European Society of Cardiology and the American College of Cardiology, Forty-ninth Scientific Sessions. Anaheim, California, March 12.

Fleming, R. M., K. M. Feldmann, and D. M. Fleming. 1999. Comparing a high-dose dipyridamole SPECT imaging protocol with dobutamine and exercise stress testing protocols. Part 3: Using dobutamine to determine lung-to-heart ratios, left ventricular dysfunction and a potential viability marker. *International J. Angiol.* 8:22–26.

———. 1998. Comparing a high-dose dipyridamole SPECT imaging protocol with dobutamine and exercise stress testing protocols. Part 2: Using high-dose dipyridamole to determine lung-to-heart ratios. *International J. Angiol.* 7:325–28.

Fleming, R. M., R. L. Kirkeeide, R. W. Smalling, et al. 1991. Patterns in visual interpretation of coronary arteriograms as detected by quantitative coronary arteriography. *J. Am. Coll. Cardiol.* 18:945–51.

Fleming, R. M., C. H. Rose, and K. M. Feldmann. 1995. Comparing a high-dose dipyridamole SPECT imaging protocol with dobutamine and exercise stress testing protocols. *Angiology* 46:547–56.

Glagov, S., E. Weisenberg, C. K. Zarins, et al. 1987. Compensatory enlargement of human atherosclerotic coronary arteries. *New Engl. J. Med.* 316: 1371–75.

Goodman, J., and L. Kirwan. 2001. Exercise-induced myocardial ischaemia in women: factors affecting prevalence. *Sports Med.* 31:235–47.

Gould, K. L. 1988. Percent coronary stenosis: battered gold standard, pernicious relic or clinical practicality? *J. Am. Coll. Cardiol.* 11:886–88.

Haack, M., A. Reichenberg, T. Kraus, et al. 2000. Effects of an intravenous catheter on the local production of cytokines and soluble cytokine receptors in healthy men. *Cytokine* 12:694–98.

Ikeda, U., Y. Maeda, and K. Shimada. 1998. Inducible nitric oxide synthetase and atherosclerosis. *Clin. Cardiol.* 21:473–76.

Inoue, T., T. Uchida, I. Yaguchi, et al. 2003. Stent-induced expression and activation of the leukocyte integrin MAC-1 is associated with neointimal thickening and restenosis. *Circulation* 107:1757–63.

Kerber, R. E., D. D. McPherson, S. J. Ross, et al. 1989. What have we learned about coronary artery disease from high-frequency epicardial echocardiography? *Int. J. Card. Imaging* 4:169–76.

Kitaoka, H., T. Yoshioka, H. Takagi, et al. 1999. Anaerobic threshold: the problem of detection of patients with heart disease. *Am. J. Med. Sports* 1:72–77.

Kuikka, J. T., O. T. Raitakari, and K. L. Gould. 2001. Imaging of the endothelial dysfunction in coronary artherosclerosis. *Eur. J. Nucl. Med.* 28:1567–78.

Kusmic, C., E. Picano, C. L. Busceti, et al. 2000. The antioxidant drug dipyridamole spares the vitamin E and thiols in red blood cells after oxidative stress. *Cardiovasc. Res.* 47:510–14.

Libby, P. 2002. Athersoclerosis: the new view. (The long-held conception of how the disease develops turns out to be wrong.) *Scientific American*, May, pp. 47–55.

Liu, J. C., D. J. Cziperle, B. Kleinman, et al. 2003. Coronary abscess: a complication of stenting. *Catheter Cardiovasc. Interv.* 58:69–71.

Llinas, R., D. Barbut, and L. R. Caplan. 2000. Neurologic complications of cardiac surgery. *Prog. Cardiovasc. Dis.* 43:101–12.

Marcus, M. L., D. G. Harrison, C. W. White, and L. F. Hiratzka. 1986. Assessing the physiological significance of coronary obstruction in man. *Can. J. Cardiol.* July (Suppl. A):195A–99A.

Marcus, M. L., D. G. Harrison, C. W. White, et al. 1988. Assessing the physiologic significance of coronary obstructions in patients: importance of diffuse undetected atherosclerosis. *Prog. Cardiovasc. Dis.* 31:39–56.

Marcus, M. L., D. J. Skorton, M. R. Johnson, et al. 1988. Visual estimates of percent diameter coronary stenosis: "a battered gold standard." *J. Am. Coll. Cardiol.* 11:882–85.

Meuwissen, M., J. J. Piek, A. C. van der Wal, et al. 2001. Recurrent unstable angina after directional coronary atherectomy is related to the extent of initial coronary plaque inflammation. *J. Am. Coll. Cardiol.* 37:1271–76.

Naghavi, M., M. Madjid, M. R. Khan, et al. 2001. New developments in the detection of vulnerable plaque. *Curr. Atheroscler. Rep.* 3:125–35.

Nissen, S. E. 2002. Who is at risk for atherosclerotic disease? Lessons from intravascular ultrasound. *Am. J. Med.* 112 (Suppl. 8A):27S–33S.

———. 1999. Shortcomings of coronary angiography and their implications in clinical practice. *Cleve. Clin. J. Med.* 66:479–485.

Nolbert, G., and B. Reichart. 2001. Cardiopulmonary bypass and cerebral injury in adults. *Shock* 16:16–19.

Rinaldi, C. A., and R. J. Hall. 2000. Myocardial stunning and hibernation in clinical practice. *International J. Clin. Pract.* 54:659–64.

Topol, E. J., and S. E. Nissen. 1995. Our preoccupation with coronary luminology. The dissociation between clinical and angiographic findings in ischemic heart disease. *Circulation* 92:2333–42.

Veillard, N. R., and F. Mach. 2002. Statins: the new aspirin? *Cell. Mol. Life Sci.* 59:1771–86.

Zarins, C. K., E. Weisenberg, G. Kolettis, et al. 1988. Differential enlargement of artery segments in response to enlarging atherosclerotic plaques. *J. Vasc. Surg.* 7:386–94.

Zir, L. M., S. W. Miller, R. E. Dinsmore, et al. 1976. Interobserver variability in coronary angiography. *Circulation* 53:627–32.

Chapters 9 and 10: The Fleming STOP INFLAMMATION NOW! Program, Phases 1 and 2

Albertazzi, P., F. Pansini, G. Bonaccorsi, et al. 1998. The effect of dietary soy supplementation on hot flashes. *Obstet. Gynecol.* 91:6–11.

Alissa, E. M., S. M. Bahijri, and G. A. Ferns. 2003. The controversy surrounding selenium and cardiovascular disease: a review of the evidence. *Med. Sci. Monit.* 9:RA9–18.

Anderson, J. W., B. M. Johnstone, and M. E. Cook-Newell. 1995. Meta-analysis of the effects of soy protein intake on serum lipids. *New Engl. J. Med.* 333:276–82.

Anderson, J. W., and A. W. Major. 2002. Pulses and lipaemia, short- and long-term effect: potential in the prevention of cardiovascular disease. *Br. J. Nutr.* 88:S263–71.

Barnard, R. J. 1991. Effects of life-style modification on serum lipids. *Arch. Intern. Med.* 151:1389–94.

Cater, N. B., and A. Garg. 2002. The effect of dietary intervention on serum lipid levels in type 2 diabetes mellitus. *Curr. Diab. Rep.* 2:289–94.

Cicero, A. F., G. Vitale, G. Savino, et al. 2003. *Panax notoginseng* (Burk.) effects on fibrinogen and lipid plasma level in rats fed on a high-fat diet. *Phytother. Res.* 17:174–78.

Czernin, J., R. J. Barnard, K. T. Sun, et al. 1995. Effect of short-term cardiovascular conditioning and low-fat diet on myocardial blood flow and flow reserve. *Circulation* 92:197–204.

Dalgard, C., A. Thuroe, B. Haastrup, et al. 2001. Saturated fat intake is reduced in patients with ischemic heart disease one year after comprehensive counseling but not after brief counseling. *J. Am. Diet. Assoc.* 101:1420–29.

Davie, S. J., B. J. Gould, and J. S. Yudkin. 1992. Effect of vitamin C on gly-cosylation of proteins. *Diabetes* 41:167–73.

Feldman, E. B. 2002. The scientific evidence for a beneficial health rela-tionship between walnuts and coronary heart disease. *J. Nutr.* 132: 1062S–1101S.

Fleming, R. M. 2003. Caloric intake, not carbohydrate or fat consumption, determines weight loss. *Am. J. Med.* 114:78.

——. 2002a. The effect of dieting on weight loss and cardiovascular disease. Forty-ninth Annual Congress of the American College of Angiology, La-haina, Maui, Hawaii, October 14.

——. 2002b. The effect of low-fat, moderate-fat and high-fat diets on weight loss and cardiovascular disease risk factors. The Asian-Pacific Scientific Forum. The Genetic Revolution: Bench to Bedside to Community. Forty-second Annual Conference on Cardiovascular Disease Epidemiol-ogy and Prevention, Honolulu, Hawaii, April 24.

——. 2000a. The clinical importance of risk factor modification: looking at both myocardial viability (MV) and myocardial perfusion imaging (MPI). *Intern. J. Angiol.* 9:55–69.

——. 2000b. The natural progression of atherosclerosis in an untreated pa-tient with hyperlipidemia: assessment via cardiac PET. *Intern. J. Angiol.* 9:70–73.

——. 1998a. Assessing PET myocardial perfusion and viability in 32 patients undergoing risk factor modification. Sixteenth World Congress of the In-ternational Society of Heart Research, Rhodes, Greece, May 27–31.

——. 1998b. Determining the outcome of risk factor modification using positron emission tomography (PET) imaging. International College of Angiology, Fortieth Annual World Congress, Lisbon, Portugal, June 28–July 3.

——. 1998a. The importance of FDG in the assessment of risk factor mod-ification outcomes. Sixteenth World Congress of the International Soci-ety of Heart Research, Rhodes, Greece, May 27–31.

——. 1995. Reducing cholesterol and triglyceride levels in both the young and elderly patient, by dietary changes: with and without hyperlipidemic medications. Seventeenth World Congress of the International Union of Angiology, the Royal Society of Medicine, London, April 3–7.

Fleming, R. M., L. Boyd, and M. Forster. 2002. Reversing heart disease in the new millennium—the Fleming Unified Theory. *Angiology* 51:617–29.

———. 2000. Unified theory approach reduces heart disease and recovers viable myocardium. Forty-second Annual World Congress, International College of Angiology, San Diego, California, June 29.

Fleming, R. M., D. M. Fleming, and R. Gaede. 1994. Hyperlipidemic elderly patients: comparing diet and drug therapy. The Council on Arteriosclerosis for the Sixty-seventh Scientific Sessions of the AHA. November:101.

Fleming, R. M., and K. Ketcham. 1993. Dietary reinforcement is an integral component of cholesterol reduction. The Council on Arteriosclerosis for the Sixty-sixth Scientific Sessions of the AHA. September:128.

Fleming, R. M., K. Ketchum, D. M. Fleming, R. Gaede. 1997. Intensive dietary counseling is a necessary adjunct to significantly increase the effectiveness of hypolipidemic medications. Fifth World Congress on Heart Failure—Mechanisms and Management, Washington, D.C., May 11–14.

———. 1996a. Assessing the independent effect of dietary counseling and hypolipidemic medications on serum lipids. *Angiology* 47:831–40.

———. 1996b. Effect of dietary counseling on hypercholesterolemia lost unless periodic counseling continues. Sixty-ninth Scientific Sessions of the American Heart Association, New Orleans, LA, November 10–13.

———. 1995a. Controlling hypercholesterolemia by diet and drug therapy in the elderly. First Annual Scientific Session on Cardiovascular Disease in the Elderly, New Orleans, March 18.

———. 1995b. Investigating differences in cholesterol and triglyceride levels as influenced by diet and hyperlipidemic medications. Forty-second Annual World Assembly of the American College of Angiology, Maui, Hawaii, October 15–20.

———. 1995c. Treating hyperlipidemia in the elderly. *Angiology* 46:1075–83.

Fleming, R. M., and D. Rater. 1993. Dietary changes without medication can equally reduce cholesterol in both the young and older patient. The

Council on Arteriosclerosis for the Sixty-sixth Scientific Sessions of the AHA. September:128.

Fleming, R. M., D. Rater, and K. Ketcham. 1993a. Reducing cholesterol and triglycerides in the elderly patient by diet alone. The Council on Arteriosclerosis for the Sixty-sixth Scientific Sessions of the AHA. September:127.

——. 1993b. Studying the effect of medications on cholesterol and triglycerides in subjects not receiving dietary counseling. The Council on Arteriosclerosis for the Sixty-sixth Scientific Sessions of the AHA. September:128.

Fukushima, M., T. Ohashi, Y. Fujiwara, et al. 2001. Cholesterol-lowering effects of maitake (*Grifola frondosa*) fiber, shiitake (*Lentinus edodus*) fiber, and enokitake (*Flammulina velutipes*) fiber in rats. *Exp. Biol. Med.* 226:758–65.

Gavagan, T. 2002. Cardiovascular disease. *Prim. Care* 29:323–38.

Geller, J., L. Sionit, C. Partido, et al. 1998. Genistein inhibits the growth of human-patient BPH and prostate cancer in histoculture. *Prostate* 34:75–79.

Gould, T. J., K. E. Bowenkamp, G. Larson, et al. 1995. Effects of dietary restriction on motor learning and cerebellar noradrenergic dysfunction in aged F344 rats. *Brain Res.* 684:150–58.

Hausman, Patricia, M.S. 1985. *The Calcium Bible.* New York: Warner Books.

Heaton, K. W., S. N. Marcus, P. M. Emmett, et al. 1988. Particle size of wheat, maize, and oat test meals: effects on plasma glucose and insulin responses and on the rate of starch digestion in vitro. *Am. J. Clin. Nutr.* 47:675–82.

Henkin, Y. 2001. Six weeks of dietary therapy for cholesterol reduction predicts long-term success. Forty-eighth Israel Heart Society, Annual Conference, Jerusalem, April 2001.

Hugh Sinclair Unit of Human Nutrition, Department of Food Sciences and Technology, University of Reading, Whiteknights. 1997. Use of manufactured foods enriched with fish oils as a means of increasing long-chain n-3 polyunsaturated fatty acid intake. *Br. J. Nutr.* 78:193–95.

Hwa, V., Y. Oh, and R. G. Rosenfeld. 1999. The insulin-like growth factor–binding protein (IGFBP) superfamily. *Endocr. Rev.* 20:761–87.

Ingram, D., K. Sanders, M. Kolybaba, et al. 1997. Case-control study of phyto-oestrogens and breast cancer. *Lancet* 350:990–94.

Jaret, P. 1999. What medical school didn't teach you about nutrition. *Hippocrates*: 33–39.

Karvonen, H. M., N. S. Tapola, M. I. Uusitupa, et al. 2002. The effect of vegetable oil–based cheese on serum total and lipoprotein lipids. *Eur. J. Clin. Nutr.* 56:1094–1101.

King, L. A., and B. R. Carr. 1999. Phytoestrogens: fact and fiction. *Patient Care*: 127–43.

Kris-Etherton, P. M., T. D. Etherton, J. Carlson, et al. 2002. Recent discoveries in inclusive food-based approaches and dietary patterns for reduction in risk for cardiovascular disease. *Curr. Opin. Lipidol.* 13:397–407.

Kullo, I. J., W. D. Edwards, and R. S. Schwartz. 1998. Vulnerable plaque: pathobiology and clinical implications. *Ann. Intern. Med.* 129:1050–60.

Lipsenthal, L., D. Ornish, and R. M. Fleming. 2000. Diets to reduce weight and CV risk: Hype or hope? Lower fat is better. American Heart Association, 73rd Scientific Session, New Orleans, November 12.

Martinez-Gonzalez, M. A., E. Fernandez-Jarne, M. Serrano-Martinez, et al. 2002. Mediterranean diet and reduction in the risk of a first acute myocardial infarction: an operational healthy dietary score. *Eur. J. Nutr.* 41:153–60.

Miyazaki, Y., H. Koyama, M. Nojiri, et al. 2002. Relationship of dietary intake of fish and non-fish selenium to serum lipids in Japanese rural coastal community. *J. Trace Elem. Med. Biol.* 16:83–90.

Mohamed-Ali, V., M. M. Gould, S. Gillies, et al. 1995. Association of proinsulin-like molecules with lipids and fibrinogen in non-diabetic subjects—evidence against a modulating role for insulin. *Diabetologia* 38:1110–16.

Ornish, D., S. E. Brown, L. W. Scherwitz, et al. 1990. Can lifestyle changes reverse coronary heart disease? The lifestyle heart trial. *Lancet* 336: 129–33.

Preuss, H. G., S. Montamarry, B. Echard, et al. 2001. Long-term effects of chromium, grape seed extract, and zinc on various metabolic parameters of rats. *Mol. Cell. Biochem.* 223:95–102.

Proceedings of the National Academy of Sciences 89, March 1992.

Proceedings of the National Academy of Sciences 90, April 1993.

Quiles, J. L., E. Martinez, S. Ibanez, et al. 2002. Aging-related tissue-specific alterations in mitochondrial composition and function are modulated by dietary fat type in the rat. *J. Bioenerg. Biomembr.* 34:517–24.

Rabbani, P. I., H. Z. Alam, S. J. Chirtel, et al. 2001. Subchronic toxicity of fish oil concentrates in male and female rats. *J. Nutr. Sci. Vitaminol.* (Tokyo) 47:201–12.

Raghuveer, G., C. A. Sinkey, C. Chenard, et al. 2001. Effect of vitamin E on resistance vessel endothelial dysfunction induced by methionine. *Am. J. Cardiol.* 88:285–90.

Rao, A. V. 2002. Lycopene, tomatoes, and the prevention of coronary heart disease. *Exp. Biol. Med.* 227:908–13.

Reichenberg, A., R. Yirmiya, A. Schuld, et al. 2001. Cytokine-associated emotional and cognitive disturbances in humans. *Arch. Gen. Psychiatry* 58:445–52.

Ryle, A. J., S. Davie, B. J. Gould, et al. 1990. A study of the effect of diet on glycosylated haemoglobin and albumin levels and glucose tolerance in normal subjects. *Diabet. Med.* 7:865–70.

Sacks, F. M., D. Ornish, B. Rosner, et al. 1985. Plasma lipoprotein levels in vegetarians. The effect of ingestion of fats from dairy products. *JAMA* 254:1337–41.

Saito, I., K. Yonemasu, and F. Inami. 2003. Association of body mass index, body fat, and weight gain with inflammation markers among rural residents in Japan. *Circ. J.* 67:323–29.

Sola, I. E., A. C. Morillas, P. S. Garzon, et al. 2002. Cardiovascular risk factors in patients with morbid obesity: weight loss influence. *Med. Clin.* 119:485–88.

Svetkey, L. P., D. Simons-Morton, W. M. Vollmer, et al. 1999. Effects of dietary patterns on blood pressure. Subgroup analysis of the Dietary Approaches to Stop Hypertension (DASH) randomized clinical trial. *Arch. Intern. Med.* 159:285–93.

Vanharanta, M., S. Voutilainen, T. H. Rissanen, et al. 2003. Risk of cardiovascular disease–related and all-cause death according to serum concentrations of enterolactone. *Arch. Intern. Med.* 163:1099–104.

Volek, J. S., A. L. Gomez, and W. J. Kraemer. 2000. Fasting lipoprotein and postprandial triacylglycerol responses to a low-carbohydrate diet supplemented with n-3 fatty acids. *J. Am. Coll. Nutr.* 19:383–91.

Weigle, D. S., D. E. Cummings, P. D. Newby, et al. 2003. Roles of leptin and ghrelin in the loss of body weight caused by a low-fat, high-carbohydrate diet. *J. Clin. Endocrinol. Metab.* 88:1577–86.

Yirmiya, R., Y. Pollak, M. Morag, et al. 2000. Illness, cytokines, and depression. *Ann. N.Y. Acad. Sci.* 917:478–87.

Warshafsky, S., R. S. Kamer, and S. L. Sivak. 1993. Effect of garlic on total serum cholesterol. A meta-analysis. *Ann. Intern. Med.* 119:599–605.

Chapter 11: The Risks of High-Protein Diets

Anderson, J. W., and R. H. Herman. 1975. Effects of carbohydrate restriction on glucose tolerance of normal men and reactive hypoglycemic patients. *Am. J. Clin. Nutr.* 28:748–55.

Araki, H. and H. Watanabe. 1983. High-risk group for benign prostatic hypertrophy. *Prostate* 4:253–64.

Cramer, Daniel, M.D., et al. 1989. Galactose consumption and metabolism in relation to the risk of ovarian cancer. *Lancet* 2:66–71.

Cheuvront, S. N. 1999. The zone diet and athletic performance. *Sports Med.* 27:213–28.

Elliott, B., H. P. Roeser, A. Warrell, et al. 1981. Effect of a high-energy, low-carbohydrate diet on serum levels of lipids and lipoproteins. *Med. J. Aust.* 1:237–40.

Fleming, R. M. 2002. The effect of high-, moderate- and low-fat diets on weight loss and cardiovascular disease risk factors. *Prev. Cardiol.* 5:110–18.

————. 2001. Obesity and related health problems are the result of too many calories and too much saturated fat regardless of the misconceptions promoted by many popular weight-loss diets. USDA research program on health and nutrition effects of popular weight-loss diets. Washington, D.C., January 11.

————. 2000. The effect of high-protein diets on coronary blood flow. *Angiology* 51:817–26.

Freeman, J. M., E. P. Vining, D. J. Pillas, et al. 1998. The efficacy of the ketogenic diet—1998: a prospective evaluation of intervention in 150 children. *Pediatrics* 102:1358–63.

Hegsted, D. M., Ph.D. 2001. Fractures, calcium and the modern diet. *Am. J. of Clin. Nutr.* 74:571–73.

Hockaday, T. D., J. M. Hockaday, J. I. Mann, et al. 1978. Prospective comparison of modified fat-high-carbohydrate with standard low-carbohydrate dietary advice in the treatment of diabetes: one year follow-up study. *Br. J. Nutr.* 39:357–62.

Hoyt, C. S., and F. A. Billson. 1977. Low-carbohydrate diet optic neuropathy. *Med. J. Aust.* 1:65–66.

Jones, D. B., R. D. Carter, and J. I. Mann. 1986. Increased arachidonic acid level in diabetic platelets following improvement in diabetic control. *Diabet. Metab.* 12:65–67.

Kennedy, E. T., S. A. Bowman, J. T. Spence, et al. 2001. Popular diets: correlation to health, nutrition, and obesity. *J. Am. Diet. Assoc.* 101:411–20.

Larosa, J. C., A. G. Fry, R. Muesing, et al. 1980. Effects of high-protein, low-carbohydrate dieting on plasma lipoproteins and body weight. *J. Am. Diet. Assoc.* 77:264–70.

Lousley, S. E., D. B. Jones, P. Slaughter, et al. 1984. High carbohydrate–high fibre diets in poorly controlled diabetes. *Diabet. Med.* 1:21–25.

Lutz, W. 1975. Pathologic liver tests during low-carbohydrate diet. *Wien Med. Wochenschr.* 125:292–95.

McDougall, John, M.D. *The McDougall Program for Women* (New York: Dutton, 2000).

McLaughlan, J. M., D. Usher, F. J. Noel, et al. 1976. Effect of a low-carbohydrate diet and alcohol on perceptual motor skill. *J. Am. Diet. Assoc.* 68:138–42.

Murphy, M. C., S. G. Isherwood, S. Sethi, et al. 1995. Postprandial lipid and hormone responses to meals of varying fat contents: modulatory role of lipoprotein lipase? *Eur. J. Clin. Nutr.* 49:578–88.

Nestle, Marion, Ph.D. 2002. *Food Politics: How the Food Industry Influences Nutrition and Health.* Berkeley: University of California Press.

Rabast, U., K. H. Vornberger, and M. Ehl. 1981. Loss of weight, sodium and water in obese persons consuming a high- or low-carbohydrate diet. *Ann. Nutr. Metab.* 25:341–49.

Rickman, F., N. Mitchell, J. Dingman, et al. 1974. Changes in serum cholesterol during the Stillman Diet. *JAMA* 228:54–58.

Rivellese, A., G. Riccardi, A. Giacco, et al. 1980. Effect of dietary fibre on glucose control and serum lipoproteins in diabetic patients. *Lancet* 2:447–50.

Rothwell, N. J., M. J. Stock, and R. S. Tyzbir. 1982. Energy balance and mitochondrial function in liver and brown fat of rats fed "cafeteria" diets of varying protein content. *J. Nutr.* 112:1663–72.

Shiell, A. W., M. Campbell-Brown, S. Haselden, et al. 2001. High-meat, low-carbohydrate diet in pregnancy: relation to adult blood pressure in the offspring. *Hypertension* 38:1282–88.

Simpson, H. C., R. D. Carter, S. Lousley, et al. 1982. Digestible carbohydrate—an independent effect on diabetic control in type 2 (non-insulin-dependent) diabetic patients? *Diabetologia* 23:235–39.

Simpson, R. W., J. I. Mann, J. Eaton, et al. 1979. Improved glucose control in maturity-onset diabetes treated with high-carbohydrate-modified fat diet. *Br. Med. J.* 1:1753–56.

Sommariva, D., L. Scotti, and A. Fasoli. 1978. Low-fat diet versus low-carbohydrate diet in the treatment of type IV hyperlipoproteinemia. *Atherosclerosis* 29:43–51.

St. Jeor, S. T., B. V. Howard, T. E. Prewitt, et al. 2001. Dietary protein and weight reduction: a statement for healthcare professionals from the

Nutrition Committee of the Council on Nutrition, Physical Activity, and Metabolism of the American Heart Association. *Circulation* 104: 1869–74.

Suh, I., K. W. Oh, K. H. Lee, et al. 2001. Moderate dietary fat consumption as a risk factor for ischemic heart disease in a population with a low-fat intake: a case-control study in Korean men. *Am. J. Clin. Nutr.* 73:722–27.

Szot, P., D. Weinshenker, J. M. Rho, et al. 2001. Norepinephrine is required for the anticonvulsant effect of the ketogenic diet. *Brain Res. Dev. Brain Res.* 129:211–14.

Ulrich, I. H., P. J. Peters, and M. J. Albrink. 1985. Effect of low-carbohydrate diets high in either fat or protein on thyroid function, plasma insulin, glucose, and triglycerides in healthy young adults. *J. Am. Coll. Nutr.* 4:451–59.

Vidon, C., P. Boucher, A. Cachefo, et al. 2001. Effects of isoenergetic high-carbohydrate compared with high-fat diets on human cholesterol synthesis and expression of key regulatory genes of cholesterol metabolism. *Am. J. Clin. Nutr.* 73:878–84.

Vogel, R. A., M. C. Corretti, and G. D. Plotnick. 1997. Effect of a single high-fat meal on endothelial function in healthy subjects. *Am. J. Cardiol.* 79:350–54.

Walker, W. J., et al. 1953. Effect of weight reduction and caloric balance on serum lipoprotein and cholesterol levels. *Am. J. Med.* 14:654–64.

Ward, G. M., R. W. Simpson, H. C. Simpson, et al. 1982. Insulin receptor binding increased by high-carbohydrate low-fat diet in non-insulin-dependent diabetes. *Eur. J. Clin. Invest.* 12:93–96.

Willett, Walter. 2001. *Eat, Drink, and Be Healthy: The Harvard Medical School Guide to Healthy Eating.* New York: Simon & Schuster.

Chapter 12: Cancer Is Also an Inflammatory Disease

Barnard, James, W. J. Aronson, C. N. Tymchuk, and T. H. Ngo. 2002. Prostate cancer: another aspect of the insulin-resistance syndrome? *Obesity Reviews* 3(4):303–8.

Calle, E. E., C. Rodriguez, K. Walker-Thurmond, et al. 2003. Overweight, obesity, and mortality from cancer in a prospective studied cohort of U.S. adults. *N. Engl. J. Med.* 348:1625–38.

Cameron, I. L., J. Munoz, C. J. Barnes, et al. 2003. High dietary level of synthetic vitamin E on lipid peroxidation, membrane fatty acid composition and cytotoxicity in breast cancer xenograft and in mouse hose tissue. *Cancer Cell Int.* 3:3.

Charlier, C., A. Albert, P. Herman, et al. 2003. Breast cancer and serum organochlorine residues. *Occup. Environ. Med.* 60:348–51.

Dreikorn, K., R. Berges, L. Pientka, et al. 2002. Phytotherapy of benign prostatic hyperplasia. Current evidence-based evaluation. *Urologe A.* 41: 447–51.

El-Bayoumy, K., J. P. Richie, T. Boyiri, et al. 2002. Influence of selenium-enriched yeast supplementation on biomarkers of oxidative damage and hormone status in healthy adult males: a clinical pilot study. *Cancer Epidemiol. Biomarkers Prev.* 11:1459–65.

Fleming, R. M. 2003a (in press). Are there differences in breast tissue as a result of hormone replacement therapy? (Submitted April 2003.) *Integrative Cancer Therapies.*

———. 2003b (in press). Do women taking hormone replacement therapy (HRT) have a higher incidence of breast cancer than women who do not? (Submitted April 2003.) *Integrative Cancer Therapies.*

———. 2003c (in press). What effect, if any, does soy protein have on breast tissue? (Submitted April 2003.) *Integrative Cancer Therapies.*

———. 2002a. Breast-enhanced scintigraphy test demonstrates improvement in breast inflammation in women consuming soy protein. *J. Nutr.* 132:575S.

———. 2002b. Mitochondrial uptake of sestamibi distinguishes between normal, inflammatory breast changes, pre-cancers and infiltrating breast cancer. *Integrative Cancer Therapies* 1:229–37.

Fleming, R. M., and W. C. Dooley. 2002. Breast-enhanced scintigraphy testing (B.E.S.T.) distinguishes between normal, inflammatory breast changes and breast cancer. A prospective analysis and comparison with mammography. *Integrative Cancer Therapies* 1:238–45.

Giovannucci, Edward, et al. 1993. A prospective study of dietary fat and risk of prostate cancer. *J. Natl. Cancer Inst.* 85(19):1571–79.

Hoshiya, Y., T. Kubota, S. W. Matsuzaki, et al. 1996. Methionine starvation modulates the efficacy of cisplatin on human breast cancer in nude mice. *Anticancer Res.* 16:3515–17.

Inoue, M., K. Tajima, and S. Tominaga. 2000. Probabilities of developing cancer over the whole life span of a Japanese. *Asian Pac. J. Cancer Prev.* 1:333–36.

Jenkins, D. J., C. W. Kendall, P. W. Connelly, et al. 2002. Effects of high- and low-isoflavone (phytoestrogen) soy foods on inflammatory biomarkers and proinflammatory cytokines in middle-aged men and women. *Metabolism* 51:919–24.

Komninou, D., A. Ayonote, J. P. Richie, et al. 2003. Insulin resistance and its contribution to colon carcinogenesis. *Exp. Biol. Med.* 228:396–405.

Le, H. T., C. M. Schaldach, G. L. Firestone, et al. 2003 (in press). Plant derived 3,3'-diindolylmethane is a strong androgen antagonist in human prostate cancer cells. *J. Biol. Chem.* 27.

Lemieux, C., F. Picard, F. Labrie, et al. 2003. The estrogen antagonist EM-652 and dehydroepiandrosterone prevent diet- and ovariectomy-induced obesity. *Obes. Res.* 11:477–90.

McTiernan, A. 2003. Behavioral risk factors in breast cancer: can risk be modified? *Oncologist* 8 (4):326–34.

Moore, M. A., and H. Tsuda. 2002. Food and play preferences—does cancer prevention require targeting the child? *Asian Pac. J. Cancer Prev.* 3:279–80.

Petridou, E., S. Kedikoglou, P. Koukoulomatis, et al. 2002. Diet in relation to endometrial cancer risk: a case-control study in Greece. *Nutr. Cancer* 44:16–22.

Rodler, I., and G. Zajkas. 2003. Healthy nutrition and the prevention of cancer. *Orv. Hetil.* 144:413–18.

Schedlich, L. J., and L. D. Graham. 2002. Role of insulin-like growth factor binding protein-3 in breast cancer cell growth. *Microsc. Res. Tech.* 59:12–22.

Sicilia, T., H. B. Niemeyer, D. M. Honig, et al. 2003. Identification and stereochemical characterization of lignans in flaxseed and pumpkin seeds. *J. Agric. Food Chem.* 51:1181–88.

Simopoulos, A. P. 2002. The importance of the ratio of omega-6/omega-3 essential fatty acids. *Biomed. Pharmacother.* 56:365–79.

Sinagra, D., C. Amato, A. M. Scarpilta, et al. 2002. Metabolic syndrome and breast cancer risk. *Eur. Rev. Med. Pharmacol. Sci.* 6:55–59.

Toniolo, P. G., et al. 1995. A prospective study of endogenous estrogens and breast cancer in postmenopausal women. *J. Natl. Cancer Inst.* 87:190–97.

Yee, D., S. Paik, G. S. Lebovic, et al. 1989. Analysis of insulin-like growth factor I gene expression in malignancy: evidence for a paracrine role in human breast cancer. *Mol. Endocrinol.* 3:509–17.

Zhou, J. R., L. Yu, Y. Zhong, et al. 2003. Soy phytochemicals and tea bioactive components synergistically inhibit androgen-sensitive human prostate tumors in mice. *J. Nutr.* 133:516–21.

Ziegler, Regina. 1996. Relative weight, weight change, height, and breast cancer risk in Asian-American women. *J. Natl. Cancer Inst.* 88:650–60.

Zumkeller, W. 2002. IGFs and IGF-binding proteins as diagnostic markers and biological modulators in brain tumors. *Expert Rev. Mol. Diagn.* 2:473–77.

Index

Baked
  Salmon, 243–44
  Squash, 225
  Sweet Potato (or Yam), 226
Balloon angioplasty, 121, 123–24
Barley, 166
  and Shiitake Soup, 232–33
Barnard, James, Dr., 197
Beans
  Adzuki, 228
  Boiled, 228–29
  and Macaroni Salad, 242–43
  Pinto, 230–31
BEST imaging, 191
Beta-carotene, 85
Beverages, 139, 164
Biaxin, 114
Bioflavonoids, 149–51
Biphosphates, 188
Blood clots, 11, 27, 63, 80–81
  and Lp(a), 99–101
Blood panel, 129–31
Blood pressure, 62–63, 128
Blueberry Crisp, 246
Boiled
  Beans, 228–29
  Brown Rice, 238
  Carrots and Parsnips, 223
Bone-density tests, 188
Bone health
  calcium sources, 189
  and exercise, 186–87
  and high-protein diets, 183–86
  and hormones, 187–88
  and pharmaceutical drugs, 188
  and salt, 188
  and vitamin D, 187
Bovine growth hormone, 103
Bowel elimination, 200
Brain chemistry changes, 68–69
BrCA1 gene, 191
Breast cancer, 200–204
Broccoli, 147–48
Broiled Whitefish, 244
Brown rice, 166
  Boiled, 238
  Pressure-cooked, 240
Brussels sprouts, 148
Buckwheat, 167
  and Bows, 238
Butkus, Dick, 17
Bypass surgery, 121, 124–26

Cabbage, 148
  with Cumin, 226
Calcium, 144–46, 183–89
The Calcium Bible (Hausman), 145
Caloric excess, 40, 102
Cancer, 54, 190–91
  diet/soy combination for, 191–204
  and exercise, 64–65, 203–4
  and homocysteine level, 90–91
Carotenoids, 88–90, 151
Carrots, 149
  Onions, and Summer Squash, Sautéed, 237
  Onions, and Summer Squash, Water-Sautéed, 225
  and Parsnips, Boiled, 223
Caspersen, Carl, Dr., 66
Cauliflower, 148
Centers for Disease Control, 46
Cheney, Dick, 16
Chest pain, 120, 128
Chickpea, Marinated Salad, 230
Chinese-Style Vegetables, 224
Chives, 149
Chlamydia pneumoniae, 112–13
Cholesterol, 3–4, 8, 177–79
  Andrew's story, 28–29
  elevation process, 29–37
  high blood, 24–26
  ideal blood level, 37–38
  Karen's story, 22–24
  lowering and reversing heart disease, 39–42
  medications for, 42–43
  -to-HDL ratio, 38–39, 178–79
  wound-clot-heart attack process, 26–28
Church, Tim, Dr., 2
Cigarettes, 39, 128
Circulation, 63
Circumflex branch, 125
Clotting. *See* Blood clots
Coffee, 29
Cold Soba Noodles with Ginger-Sesame Sauce, 241
Collard greens, 148
Comfort foods, 140–46
Complement, 12, 25
Complex carbohydrates, 56–57
Condiments, 157, 223
Coronary
  arteries, 125
  bypass surgery, 121, 124–26

Corticosteroids, 188
COX–2, 28
Cramer, Daniel, Dr., 185
Cravings (food), 50–51
C-reactive protein, 14–15, 37, 61–62, 100–101, 130
Cruciferous vegetables, 147–48, 198
  recipes, 225–28
Cucumber, Pressed Salad, 236
Cytokines, 11, 111, 143

Daikon Radish
  Salad, 226
  with Shoyu, 227
Dairy products, 103–4, 140, 163
Dancing, 74–75
Dessert recipes, 234–35, 245–46
Diabetes, 128
  destruction of body from, 53–54
  and exercise, 64
  Type 1, 52
  Type 2, 52–53
  weight gain and insulin resistance, 51–52
Diabetes Prevention Program, 64
Diagnosis, 127–32
Diet
  AHA, 173, 175
  anti-cancer, 191–204
  Asian, 194, 200
  Fleming
    Phase 1, 136–41
    Phase 2, 161–70
    vs. high-protein, 171–82
  high-fiber, 40
  high-protein, 80–82, 171–82
  and homocysteine, 79–83
  inadequacy of changes in, 19
  plant-based, 181–82, 198–99
  Western, 6, 17–18, 48–50, 56, 204
Dihydrotestosterone, 194–95
Dining-out guidelines, 161–62
Doppler ultrasound, 129
Dressings, 233–34, 242–45
Duncan, J. J., 64
Dysrhythmia, 128

Echocardiogram, 128–29
Edamame, 154
Ejection fraction, 125
Endorphins, 69
Energy levels, 143

Essential fatty acids, 34, 117–18
Estradiol, 201
Estriol, 201
Estrogen, 54, 97, 147, 187, 194–97, 200
  plant, 152
Estrone, 201
Ettinger, Bruce, Dr., 96
European Journal of Clinical Nutrition, 54
Exercise, 10–11, 21, 61–62, 143
  becoming your best self, 69–72
  and bone health, 186–87
  diabetes, insulin, and inflammation, 64
  fibrinogen and blood clots, 63
  and Fleming Program, 72–75
    Phase 1, 157–58
  fun and consistency in, 76
  going slowly, 63–64
  high blood pressure and inflammation, 62–63
  for immune-system boost and cancer, 64–65, 193, 203–4
  and living longer, 65–66
  patterns, 128
  positive brain chemistry changes from, 68–69
  and preference for healing foods, 66–68

Fasting glucose, 130
Fats, 29, 51
  hydrogenated, 30
  monounsaturated, 34–35
  polyunsaturated, 30, 33–34
  saturated, 30, 40
Fatty streak, 3, 26
Fiber, 151–52, 192, 199–200
Fibrinogen, 11, 63, 95–96, 130, 143, 180
  lowering, 100–101
Fish, 169
  recipes, 243–44
Flaxseeds, 117–18, 138, 155–56, 163
Fleming Program, 40–41, 105
  for cancer treatment, 190–205
  exercise portion, 72–76
  menus for, 207–18
  overview, 6–7, 19–21
  Phase 1, 134–60
  Phase 1a, 159–60
  Phase 2, 161–70
Flour products, 140
Foam cells, 25
Folic acid, 81, 138